Care in Mental Health–Substance Use

MENTAL HEALTH–SUBSTANCE USE

Care in Mental Health–Substance Use

Edited by

DAVID B COOPER

Sigma Theta Tau International: The Honor Society of Nursing Award
Outstanding Contribution to Nursing Award
Editor-in-Chief, Mental Health and Substance Use
Author/Writer/Editor

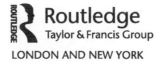

Routledge
Taylor & Francis Group

LONDON AND NEW YORK

First published 2011 by Radcliffe Publishing Ltd

Published 2018 by Routledge

2 Park Square, Milton Park, Abingdon, Oxfordshire OX14 4RN

711 Third Avenue, New York, NY 10017

Electronic catalogue and worldwide online ordering facility.

British Library Cataloguing in Publication Data

A catalogue record for this book is available from the British Library.

ISBN-13: 978-1-138-45008-0 (hbk)
ISBN-13: 978-1-84619-343-9 (pbk)

Typeset by Pindar NZ, Auckland, New Zealand

Contents

Preface

Approximately six years ago Phil Cooper, then an MSc student, was searching for information on mental health–substance use. At that time, there was one journal and few published papers. This led to the launch of the journal *Mental Health and Substance Use: dual diagnosis*, published by Taylor & Francis International. To launch the journal, and debate the concerns and dilemmas of psychological, physical, social, legal and spiritual professionals, Phil organised a conference for Suffolk Mental Health NHS Trust and Taylor & Francis. The response was excellent. An occurring theme was that more information, knowledge and skills were needed – driven by education and training.

Discussion with international professionals indicated a need for this type of educational information and guidance, in this format, and a proposal was submitted for one book. The single book progressed to become a series of six! The concept is that each book will follow on from the other to build a sound basis – as far as is possible – about the important approaches to mental health–substance use. The aim is to provide a 'how to' series that will be interactive with case studies, reflective study and exercises – you, as individuals and professionals, will decide if this has been achieved.

So, why do we need to know about mental health–substance use? International concerns related to interventions, and the treatment of people experiencing mental health–substance use problems, are frequently reported. These include:

➤ 'the most challenging clinical problem that we face'[1]
➤ 'substance misuse is usual rather than exceptional amongst people with severe mental health problems'[2]
➤ 'Mental health and substance use problems affect every local community throughout America'[3]
➤ 'The existence of psychiatric comorbidities in young people who abuse alcohol is common, especially for conditions such as depression, anxiety, bipolar disorder, conduct disorder and attention-deficit/hyperactivity disorder'[4]
➤ 'Mental and neurological disorders such as depression, schizophrenia, epilepsy and substance abuse . . . cause immense suffering for those affected, amplify people's vulnerability and can lead individuals into a life of poverty'.[5]

There is a need to appreciate that mental health–substance use is now a concern for us all. This series of books will bring together what is known (to some), and what is not (to some). If undertaken correctly, and you, the reader will be the judge – and those individuals you come into contact with daily will be the final judges – each book will build on the other and be of interest for the new, and the not so new, professional.

The desire to provide services that facilitate best practice for mental health–substance use is not new. The political impetus for this approach to succeed now exists. We, the professionals, need to seize on this momentum. We need to bring about the much-needed change for the individual who experiences our interventions and treatment, be that political will because of a perceived financial benefit or, as we would hope, the need to provide therapeutic interventions for the individual. Whatever the motive, now is the time to grasp the initiative.

Before we (the professionals) can practise, research, educate, manage, develop or purchase services, we must commence with knowledge. From that, we begin to understand. We commence using our new-found skills. We progress to developing the ability to examine practice, to put concepts together, to make valid judgements. We achieve this level of expertise though education, training and experience. Sometimes, we can use our own life experiences to enhance our skills. But knowledge must come first, though is often relegated to last! Professionals (from health, social, spiritual and legal backgrounds) – be they students, practitioners, researchers, educators, managers, service developers or purchasers – are all 'professionals' (in the eye of the individual we meet professionally), though each has differing depths of knowledge, skills and expertise.

What we need to remember is that the individual (those we offer care to), family and carers bring their own knowledge, skills and life experiences – some developed from dealing with ill health. The individual experiences the illness, lives with it, manages it – daily. Therefore, to bring the two together, individual and professional, to make interventions and treatment outcome effective, to meet whatever the individual feels is acceptable to his or her needs, requires mutual understanding and respect. The professional's skills and expertise '*are founded on nothing less than their complete and perfect acceptance of one, by another*'.[6]

David B Cooper
January 2011

REFERENCES

1 Appleby L. *The National Service Framework for Mental Health: five years on*. London: Department of Health; 2004. Available at: www.dh.gov.uk/prod_consum_dh/groups/dh_digitalassets/@dh/@en/documents/digitalasset/dh_4099122.pdf (accessed 29 August 2010).

2 Department of Health. *Mental Health Policy Implementation Guide: dual diagnosis good practice guide*. London: Department of Health; 2002. Available at: www.nmhdu.org.uk/silo/files/mental-health-policy--implementation-guide.pdf (accessed 29 August 2010).

3 Substance Abuse and Mental Health Service Administration. *Results from the 2008 National Survey on Drug Use and Health*. 2008. Available at: www.oas.samhsa.gov/nsduh/2k8nsduh/2k8Results.cfm (accessed 2 August 2010).

4 Australian Government. *Australian Guidelines to Reduce Health Risks from Drinking Alcohol*.

2009. Available at: www.nhmrc.gov.au/publications/synopses/ds10syn.htm (accessed 29 August 2010).

5 World Health Organization. *Mental Health Improvements for Nations Development: the WHO MIND Project.* World Health Organization; 2008. Available at: www.who.int/mental_health/policy/en (accessed 29 August 2010).

6 Thompson F. *Lark Rise to Candleford: a trilogy.* London: Penguin Modern Classics; 2009.

About the Mental Health–Substance Use series

The six books in this series are:
1 *Introduction to Mental Health–Substance Use*
2 *Developing Services in Mental Health–Substance Use*
3 *Responding in Mental Health–Substance Use*
4 *Intervention in Mental Health–Substance Use*
5 *Care in Mental Health–Substance Use*
6 *Practice in Mental Health–Substance Use*

The series is not merely for mental health professionals but also for the substance use professionals. It is not a question of 'them' (the substance use professional) teaching 'them' (the mental health professional). It is about sharing knowledge, skills and expertise. We are equal. We learn from each fellow professional, for the benefit of those whose lives we touch. The rationale is that to maintain clinical excellence, we need to be aware of the developments and practices within mental health and substance use. Then, we make informed choices; we take best practice, and apply this to our professional role.[1]

Generically, the series Mental Health–Substance Use concentrates on concerns, dilemmas and concepts specifically interrelated, as a collation of problems that directly or indirectly influence the life and well-being of the individual, family and carers. Such concerns relate not only to the individual but also to the future direction of practice, education, research, service development, interventions and treatment. While presenting a balanced view of what is best practice today, the books aim to challenge concepts and stimulate debate, exploring all aspects of the development in treatment, intervention and care responses, and the adoption of research-led best practice. To achieve this, they draw from a variety of perspectives, facilitating consideration of how professionals meet the challenges now and in the future. To accomplish this we have assembled leading, international professionals to provide insight into current thinking and developments, from a variety of perspectives, related to the many varying and diverse needs of the individual, family and carers experiencing mental health–substance use.

REFERENCE

1 Cooper DB. Editorial: decisions. *Mental Health and Substance Use.* 2010; **3**: 1–3.

About the editor

David B Cooper
Sigma Theta Tau International: The Honor Society of Nursing Award
Outstanding Contribution to Nursing Award
Editor-in-Chief: *Mental Health and Substance Use*
Author/Writer/Editor

The editor welcomes approaches and feedback, positive and/or negative.

David has specialised in mental health and substance use for over 30 years. He has worked as a practitioner, manager, researcher, author, lecturer and consultant. He has served as editor, or editor-in-chief, of several journals, and is currently editor-in-chief of *Mental Health and Substance Use*. He has published widely and is *credited with enhancing the understanding and development of community detoxification for people experiencing alcohol withdrawal*' (Nursing Council on Alcohol; Sigma Theta Tau International citations). Seminal work includes *Alcohol Home Detoxification and Assessment* and *Alcohol Use*, both published by Radcliffe Publishing, Oxford.

List of contributors

CHAPTER 2   Kim Moore
Nurse Consultant (Dual Diagnosis)
Eastern and Coastal Kent Region
Honorary Lecturer
Department of Modernisation and Nursing
Kent and Medway Mental Health and Social Care Partnership Trust
Canterbury Christ Church University
Mental Health and Social Care Studies
Herne Bay, Kent
England

Kim is a registered mental health nurse working in substance misuse and mental health settings for over 20 years in Australia and the United Kingdom. She has a special interest in dual diagnosis, working to develop specialist services and practice in London and Kent. She works within a community mental health team and continues to be involved in delivering dual diagnosis training for postgraduate education at Christ Church University as a Consultant Nurse practitioner.

CHAPTER 3   Shona McIntosh
Lead Consultant Clinical Psychologist/Consultant Clinical Neuropsychologist
Tayside and East Central Scotland Substance Misuse Managed Care Network
Substance Misuse Psychology Services, ECSAS MCN
Perth, Scotland

Shona trained as a Clinical Psychologist in Wessex specialising in neuropsychology, psychodynamic and systemic psychotherapies. In addition, she trained in Group Analysis completing her Advanced Training in 2007. Shona has worked across services in England and Scotland including primary care, community mental health, neuropsychology and substance misuse. For some years, Shona was a researcher with the University of Southampton. She was Senior Clinical Tutor for Edinburgh University's Doctorate in Clinical Psychology. She has chaired and held posts in several British Psychological Society's committees and remains active in the governance of Clinical Psychologists' training throughout the UK.

CHAPTER 4   Alison Sadler
Clinical Manager
Sheffield Mind
Sheffield, Yorkshire
England

Alison spent many years in nursing before taking up a career in counselling and working as a British Association of Counselling and Psychotherapy accredited counsellor in both the health service and the voluntary sector. Alison has been in the field of substance misuse for the past ten years, first working with substance users and then moving on to work with their families. As Project Manager at RODA (Relatives of Drug Abusers), Alison helped develop a small charity into an organisation able to manage a commissioned contract for family support. Alison recently moved to the post of Clinical Manager at Sheffield Mind.

CHAPTER 5   Professor Charlotte de Crespigny
Professor of Drug and Alcohol Nursing and Joint Chair
Drug and Alcohol Services South Australia and the University of Adelaide
Adelaide, South Australia
Australia

Charlotte is a registered nurse working in the drug and alcohol field as a clinician, educator and researcher since 1988. Charlotte's current research interests include: systems of care; alcohol, drug and mental health comorbidity; coordinated Aboriginal mental health care; Aboriginal people's use of over-the-counter analgesics; women, alcohol and licensed premises; social drinking in context; heatwave and the impact on vulnerable people with mental health and substance use conditions. Charlotte works in partnership with other researchers and practitioners from varying health fields including mental health, public health, health economics and Aboriginal health. She is committed to translating research findings into everyday healthcare, including clinical practice, health promotion and community and professional education. Charlotte has many journal publications, best practice guidelines and chapters in texts.

Scekar Valadian
Senior Project Officer
Aboriginal Community Team
Drug and Alcohol Service South Australia
161 Greenhill Road
Parkside, South Australia
Australia

Scekar is a senior Aboriginal project officer. He has worked for over 12 years in the drug and alcohol field as a counsellor and educator, with a special interest in ensuring cultural respectful services across the drug and alcohol field. Scekar has been a significant leader in the field through his commitment to advancing knowledge about the various alcohol and drug issues pertinent to Indigenous people. This has been exemplified through his involvement in the national development and implementation of the *National Alcohol Treatment Guidelines for Indigenous Australians*. For over two years, Scekar worked alongside Charlotte in the provision of workshops across rural and remote Australia for Indigenous and non-indigenous health professionals to enable them to make best use of the guidelines. In 2007 Scekar and Charlotte were joint keynote speakers at the 2007 Australian Professional Society of Alcohol and Drugs (APSAD) and Cutting Edge Conference – *Two Nations – 10 Cultures?* in Auckland, New Zealand.

CHAPTER 6   Ian Wilson
Clinical Teaching Fellow, University of Manchester
Dual Diagnosis Trainer/Clinical Nurse
School of Nursing, Midwifery and Social Work
Manchester Health and Social Care Trust
Manchester, England

Ian is a mental health nurse. Ian has a particular interest in the application of evidence-based interventions for people with complex mental health needs and substance misuse problems, working with carers of 'dually diagnosed' clients and addressing the training requirements of a wide range of workers who come into contact with clients exhibiting complex needs.

CHAPTER 7   David Watkins
Families where a Parent has a Mental Illness (FaPMI) Coordinator
Integrated Primary Mental Health Service
Northeast Health Wangaratta
Wangaratta, Victoria
Australia

David is a registered psychiatric nurse. Since 1983, David has worked in a number of clinical and managerial roles in mental health services in Victoria, Australia. David's experience is broad and formal interests involve the scope of academic, clinical and research domains in psychiatric/mental health nursing, problem gambling, health services research and evaluation and public health issues, particularly as they relate to populations with mental health problems. David has published and presented in his fields of interest at a range of national and international conference forums. Most recently, David has worked in rural Victoria as the coordinator of Families where a Parent has a Mental Illness (FaPMI). In this role, David performs service development tasks within the Northeast Victorian Area Mental Health Service. In addition, he engages with the wider network of services through developing and delivering a range of training packages; policy development; and enhancement of the capacity of the mental health service workforce.

Francis McCormick
State-wide Coordinator for Families where a Parent has a Mental Illness (FaPMI)

The Bouverie Centre – Victoria's Family Institute
Brunswick
Melbourne, Victoria
Australia

Francis has worked in psychiatry for over 25 years, in inpatient and community-based services in public mental health and in general practice settings. He has 15 years' experience in child and adolescent mental health, with a special interest in family therapy and adolescents with high-risk issues. Francis has contributed to a number of new initiatives in mental health, including mental health consultancy to youth services, and over the past four years in the area of FaPMI. Currently, as the FaPMI coordinator in a rural region of Victoria, Australia, Francis focuses on improving workforce capacity to respond better to families. He also works part-time as a clinician providing psychologically focused therapies.

Rosemary Cuff
Families where a Parent has a Mental Illness (FaPMI) Coordinator
Psychiatric Services
Bendigo Health
Bendigo, Victoria
Australia

Rose qualified as an occupational therapist in England in 1980 and since 1986 has worked in child, adolescent and adult mental health services in Australia. Since 1995, Rose has worked in Melbourne and focused specifically on addressing the support needs for families where a parent has a mental illness, through direct clinical practice, listening to families' stories and developing resources. Since 2007, Rose has worked in a more strategic role as the State-wide FaPMI Coordinator. This is a service development strategy with recurrent funding aimed at improving service outcomes for FaPMI across mental health and community organisations. Rose is a passionate advocate for children, young people and families and in a related role is involved in establishing a foundation to provide peer support activities for these families across Victoria.

CHAPTER 8   Professor Brian R Rush
Senior Scientist, Centre for Addiction and Mental Health
Co-Director, Health Systems Research and Consulting Unit
Centre for Addiction and Mental Health
Professor, Department of Psychiatry, University of Toronto
Associate Professor, Dalla Lana School of Public Health, University of Toronto
Toronto, Ontario
Canada

Brian holds a PhD in epidemiology and biostatistics and has worked for 33 years in a research and evaluation capacity in the substance abuse, problem gambling and mental health fields. Brian's research and development portfolio includes the field of co-occurring disorders with an emphasis on epidemiology in general and service populations, service and system level integration, and screening and assessment tools.

Dr Saulo Castel
Director, Inpatient Unit
Department of Psychiatry, Sunnybrook Health Sciences Centre
Director, Medical Education and Research
Ontario Shores, Centre for Mental Health Sciences
Assistant Professor, Department of Psychiatry
University of Toronto
Toronto, Ontario
Canada

Saulo graduated in medicine with specialisation in psychiatry and obtained a PhD in addictions at the University of Sao Paulo, Brazil. He did a postdoctoral fellowship on concurrent disorders at the Centre of Addiction and Mental Health, University of Toronto. After five years working with patients with severe mental illnesses in a psychiatric hospital, Saulo currently works with inpatients in an acute psychiatric ward in a teaching hospital, where he also supervises residents and medical students. Saulo's research interests and projects are in concurrent disorders, patient safety, guideline implementation and health systems' research in mental health.

CHAPTER 9 **Michael Adams**
Community Mental Health Nurse
Swansea Assertive Outreach Service
Clydach Hospital
Clydach
Swansea, Wales

Mick has 25 years' experience of working within the field. Mick currently practises within a Welsh assertive outreach service, where concurrent mental health–substance use problems amongst the users of the service are commonplace. Mick has previously held a variety of community posts and has experience of working as a tutor-practitioner in Swansea University teaching and publishing on mental health and substance use related issues.

Gemma Stacey-Emile
Team Leader – Alcohol Services
Hywel Dda Health Board
West Wales Substance Misuse Service
Milford Haven
Pembrokeshire, Wales

Gemma has worked for the service for nine years. Gemma qualified as a registered mental health nurse in 1995, and is currently studying for her MSc in healthcare management at Swansea University. Gemma has been active in the joint development of alcohol services across Pembrokeshire, Carmarthenshire and Ceredigion and has an excellent working relationship with colleagues specifically from social care and housing and prison.

CHAPTER 10   Karl V Robins

Senior Lecturer
Faculty of Health and Social Care
Department of Mental Health and Learning Disabilities
Anglia Ruskin University
Chelmsford, Essex
England

Karl has a background in community mental health nursing and a specialist interest in the problematic use of drugs and alcohol, and specifically dual diagnosis. Karl has incorporated collaborative approaches including motivational interviewing and solution focused brief therapy into his work. He has a particular interest in developing solution focused approaches in educational as well as clinical environments. Karl primarily lectures on pre-registration nursing, dual diagnosis, health psychology and solution focused brief therapy.

David A Hingley
Mental Health Nurse
Senior Lecturer
Faculty of Health and Social Care
Department of Mental Health and Learning Disabilities
Anglia Ruskin University
Chelmsford, Essex
England

David has used solution focused brief therapy in his practice since 1995, and now uses solution focused principles and ideas in higher education. Current interests include ideas of recovery in mental health, true collaborative practice, working with families and carers, and working with people who feel that suicide is their only choice. In 2001, he trained as a solution focused team coach at the Helsinki Brief Therapy Institute, and has published on recovery and the links between recovery and solution focused brief therapy.

CHAPTER 11   Michael Fitzsimmons

Psychological Therapist
Early Intervention Service
Lancashire Care Trust
Blackburn, Lancashire
England

Mike has worked in community mental healthcare for 20 years and has for the past six years been involved in developing therapeutic approaches for people with psychosis and comorbid substance misuse with colleagues at the University of Manchester. Mike is a member of the international Motivational Interviewing Network of Trainers.

Professor Christine Barrowclough
Professor of Clinical Psychology
School of Psychological Sciences
University of Manchester
Manchester, England

Christine has over 25 years' clinical and research experience in the development and evaluation of psychological treatments for psychosis and has published widely in this field. In the last ten years along with colleagues in Manchester, Christine has developed and published work describing the evaluation of specialised approaches for working with people with psychosis and comorbid substance misuse.

CHAPTER 12   Derek Tobin
Team Manager
COMPASS programme
Handsworth
Birmingham, England

Derek is team manager of the COMPASS programme and has worked with people with combined mental health and substance problems for ten years. His background is in mental health nursing with a range of experience working in various mental health settings. He has been closely involved in the evaluation of cognitive behavioural integrated treatment (C-BIT) within assertive outreach teams. He has also overseen the development of C-BIT in early intervention services. Derek remains at the forefront of service development for mental health and substance use in Birmingham and Solihull Mental Health Foundation Trust.

CHAPTER 13   Dr Cynthia MA Geppert
Chief Consultant Psychiatry and Ethics New Mexico Veterans Affairs Health Care System
Associate Professor, Department of Psychiatry
Director of Ethics Education, University of New Mexico School of Medicine
Albuquerque, New Mexico
USA

Cynthia is board certified in general psychiatry, psychosomatic medicine, and hospice and palliative medicine, certified by the American Board of Addiction Medicine and holds credentials in pain management. She specialises in the treatment of patients with medical illnesses, co-occurring disorders, chronic pain and in palliative care. Cynthia teaches, writes and conducts research in the fields of consultation psychiatry, clinical ethics, spirituality, medical education, addiction and psychopharmacology.

Dr Kenneth Minkoff
Clinical Assistant Professor of Psychiatry
Harvard Medical School
Senior Systems Consultant, Zia Partners, San Rafael, California
Acton, Massachusetts
USA

Kenneth is a board-certified psychiatrist with a certificate of additional qualifications in addiction psychiatry. A dedicated community psychiatrist, Kenneth is recognised as one of the nation's leading experts on integrated treatment of individuals with co-occurring psychiatric and substance disorders, and on the development of integrated systems of care for such individuals, through the implementation of a national consensus best practice model for systems design: the Comprehensive Continuous Integrated System of Care (CCISC), referenced in SAMHSA's Report to Congress on Co-occurring Disorders (2002). In addition, Kenneth is a member of the Board of Directors of the American Association of Community Psychiatrists and is Chair of the Health Care Policy Committee combining his expertise in dual diagnosis and managed care. Kenneth was panel chair for CMHS Managed Care Initiative report entitled: *Co-Occurring Psychiatric and Substance Disorders in Managed Care Systems: standards of care, practice guidelines, workforce competencies, and training curricula* (1998) (*see* www.med.upenn.edu/cmhpsr). Kenneth's major professional activity is the provision of training and consultation on clinical services and systems design for individuals and families with mental health and substance use disorders. With his consulting partner, Christie A Cline, MD, MBA (former Medical Director for the Behavioral Health Services Division of the New Mexico Department of Health), Kenneth has developed a systems change toolkit for CCISC implementation (*see* www.zialogic.org). Kenneth and/or Dr Cline are currently providing (or have provided) consultation for CCISC implementation in over 35 states and four Canadian provinces, working with every aspect of state-level systems, county-level systems, tribal entities and providers of all types.

CHAPTER 14   Reverend Doctor Je Kan Adler-Collins
Associate Professor of Nursing, Health Promotion Centre; Research Fellow, Centre of Gender Studies, Khon Kaen University, Thailand
President, Non-Profit Organisation: Integrative Care Education Research Association Japan
Health Promotion Centre
Fukuoka Prefectural University
Tagawa City
Japan

Je Kan qualified as an Registered Nurse (RN), and Medical Emergency Response Team (MERT) in the British Army. He became a Buddhist monk of Shingon Shu in

Japan in 1995. Je Kan was awarded his PGCE(FE) in 1998, MA in education 2000, and PhD in education 2007. Je Kan moved to Japan in 2000 where he built a temple, school, centre and hospice. He is an Associate Professor of Nursing at Fukuoka Prefectural University. In 2009, he became Director of Education for the Japanese Holistic Nursing Association. In 2010, Je Kan became President of a new non-profit organisation, Integrative Care Education and Research Association of Japan.

CHAPTER 15   **Peter Athanasos**
Lecturer
Coordinator of Addiction and Mental Health Programs
Discipline of Nursing
Royal Adelaide Hospital
University of Adelaide
Adelaide, South Australia
Australia

Peter is a lecturer and the author and coordinator of addiction and mental health programmes at the University of Adelaide. His PhD concerned pain management in opioid-maintained patients. Peter's greatest research interest is the effect of substance use on coexisting disorders such as mental health, pain and other pathophysiology. He has authored a textbook on addiction and a number of chapters and articles in these areas.

Dr Rose Neild
Lead Clinician Medical Detoxification Service
Pregnancy and Parental Service
Waitemata DHB (Auckland) New Zealand
Community Alcohol and Drug Centre
Pt Chevalier, Auckland
New Zealand

Rose is the New Zealand branch chair of the Chapter of Addiction Medicine and represents New Zealand on the council of the Australian Professional Society on Alcohol and Other Drugs. Rose has experience of working in alcohol and other drug services in New Zealand and Australia. Rose has a particular interest in working with women with substance use disorders especially those who are pregnant or parenting and this has developed over recent times into a wider interest in inclusive practice – working with families and partners. Other interest areas include physical and psychiatric comorbidities with dependence in both clinical and public health arenas.

Professor Charlotte de Crespigny (*also* Chapter 5)

Dr Lynette Cusack
Research Fellow (Population Health)
School of Nursing and Midwifery

Faculty of Health Science
Flinders University
Adelaide, South Australia
Australia

Lynette holds a Postdoctoral Research Fellow (Population Health) position, and is a member of the Board of the Flinders University Research Centre for Disaster Resilience and Health. Lynette previously worked in the alcohol and other drug field for over 14 years in an executive role with the Drug and Alcohol Services South Australia, which is a State government organisation.

USEFUL CONTACTS

Jo Cooper
Former Macmillan Clinical Nurse Specialist in Palliative Care
Horsham, West Sussex
England

Jo spent 16 years in specialist palliative care, initially working in a hospice inpatient unit, then 12 years as a Macmillan Clinical Nurse Specialist. She gained a Diploma in Oncology at Addenbrooke's Hospital, Cambridge, and a BSc (Hons) in palliative nursing at The Royal Marsden, London, and an Award in Specialist Practice. Jo edited *Stepping into Palliative Care* (Radcliffe Medical Press; 2000) and the second edition of *Stepping into Palliative Care*, Books 1 and 2 (Radcliffe Publishing; 2006). Jo has been involved in teaching for many years and her specialist subjects include management of complex pain and symptoms, terminal agitation, communication at the end of life, therapeutic relationships and breaking bad news.

Terminology

Whenever possible, the following terminology has been applied. However, in certain instances, when referencing a study and/or specific work(s), when an author has made a specific request, or for the purpose of additional clarity, it has been necessary to deviate from this applied 'norm'.

MENTAL HEALTH–SUBSTANCE USE

Considerable thought has gone in to the use of terminology within these texts. Each country appears to have its own terms for the person experiencing mental health and substance use problems – terms that includes words such as dual diagnosis, coexisting, co-occurring, and so on. We talk about the same thing but use differing professional jargon. The decision was set at the outset to use one term that encompasses mental health *and* substance use problems: *mental health–substance use*. One scholar suggested that such a term implies that both can exist separately, while they can also be linked.[1]

SUBSTANCE USE

Another challenge was how to term 'substance use'. There are a number of ways: abuse, misuse, dependence, addiction. The decision is that within these texts we use the term *substance use* to encompass all (unless specific need for clarity at a given point). It is imperative the professional recognises that while we may see another person's 'substance use' as misuse or abuse, the individual experiencing it may not deem it to be anything other than 'use'. Throughout, we need to be aware that we are working alongside unique individuals. Therefore, we should be able to meet the individual where he/she is.

ALCOHOL, PRESCRIBED DRUGS, ILLICIT DRUGS, TOBACCO OR SUBSTANCES

Throughout this book *substance* includes alcohol, prescribed drugs, illicit drugs and tobacco, unless specific need for clarity at a given point.

PROBLEM(S), CONCERNS AND DILEMMAS OR DISORDERS

The terms *problem(s)*, *concerns and dilemmas* and *disorders* can be used interchangeably, as stated by the author's preference. However, where possible, the term 'problem(s)' or 'concerns and dilemmas' had been adopted as the preferred choice.

INDIVIDUAL, PERSON, PEOPLE

There seems to be a need to label the individual – as a form of recognition! Sometimes the label becomes more than the person! 'Alan is schizophrenic' – thus it is Alan, rather than an illness that Alan lives with. We refer to patients, clients, service users, customers, consumers, and so on. Yet, we feel affronted when we are addressed as anything other than what we are – individuals! We need to be mindful that every person we see during our professional day is an individual – unique. Symptoms are in many ways similar (e.g. delusions, hallucinations), some need interventions and treatments are similar (e.g. specific drugs, psychotherapy techniques), but people are not. Alan may experience an illness labelled schizophrenia, and so may John, Beth and Mary, and you or I. However, each will have his/her own unique experiences – and life. None will be the same. To keep this constantly in the mind of the reader, throughout the book series we shall refer to the *individual*, *person* or *people* – just like us, but different to us by their uniqueness.

PROFESSIONAL

We are all professionals, whether students, nurses, doctors, social workers, researchers, clinicians, educationalists, managers, service developers, religious ministers – and so on. However, the level of expertise may vary from one professional to another. We are also individuals. There is a need to distinguish between the person with a mental health–substance use problem and the person interacting professionally (at whatever level) with that individual. To acknowledge and to differentiate between those who experience – in this context – and those who intervene, we have adopted the term *professional*. It is indicative that we have had, or are receiving, education and training related specifically to help us (the professionals) meet the needs of the individual. We may or may not have experienced mental health–substance use problems but we have some knowledge that may help the individual – an expertise to be shared. We have a specific knowledge that, hopefully, we wish to use to offer effective intervention and treatment to another human being. It is the need to make a clear differential, for the reader, that forces the use of 'professional' over 'individual' to describe our role – our input into another person's life.

REFERENCE

1 Barker P. Personal communication; 2009.

Cautionary note

Wisdom and compassion should become the dominating influence that guide our thoughts, our words, and our actions.[1]

Never presume that what you say is understood. It is essential to check understanding, and what is expected of the individual and/or family, with each person. Each person needs to know what he/she can expect from you, and other professionals involved in his/her care, at each meeting. Jargon is a professional language that excludes the individual and family. Never use it in conversation with the individual, unless requested to do so; it is easily misunderstood.

Remember, we all, as individuals, deal with life differently. It does not matter how many years we have spent studying human behaviour, listening and treating the individual and family. We may have spent many hours exploring with the individual his/her anxieties, fears, doubts, concerns and dilemmas, and the illness experience. Yet, we do not know what that person really feels, how he/she sees life and ill health. We may have lived similar lives, experienced the same illness but the individual will always be unique, each different from us, each independent of our thoughts, feelings, words, deeds and symptoms, each with an individual experience.

REFERENCE

1 Matthieu Ricard. As cited in: Föllmi D, Föllmi O. *Buddhist Offerings 365 Days*. London: Thames & Hudson; 2003.

Acknowledgements

I am grateful to all the contributors for having the faith in me to produce a valued text and I thank them for their support and encouragement. I hope that faith proves correct. Thank you to those who have commented along the way, and whose patience has been outstanding. Thank you to Jo Cooper, who has been actively involved with this project throughout – supporting, encouraging, listening and participating in many practical ways. Jo is my rock who looks after me during my physical health problems, and I am eternally grateful.

Many people have helped me along my career path and life – too many to name individually. Most do not even know what impact they have had on me. Some, however, require specific mention. These include Larry Purnell, a friend and confidant who has taught me never to presume – while we are all individuals with individual needs, we deserve equality in all that we meet in life. Thanks to Martin Plant (who sadly died in March 2010), and Moira Plant, who always encouraged and offered genuine support. Phil and Poppy Barker, who have taught me that it is OK to express how I feel about humanity – about people, and that there is another way through the entrenched systems in health and social care. Keith Yoxhall, without whose guidance back in the 1980s I would never have survived my 'Colchester work experience' and the dark times of institutionalisation, or had the privilege to work alongside the few professionals fighting against the 'big door'. He taught me that there was a need for education and training, and that this should be ongoing – also that the person in hospital or community experiencing our care sees us as 'professional' – we should make sure we act that way. Thank you to Phil Cooper, who brought the concept of this book series to me via a conference to launch the journal *Mental Health and Substance Use: dual diagnosis*, of which he was editor. It was then I realised that despite all the talk over too many years of my professional life, there was still much to be done for people experiencing mental health–substance use problems. Phil is a good debater, friend and reliable resource for me – thank you.

To Gillian Nineham of Radcliffe Publishing, my sincere thanks. Gillian had faith in this project from the outset and in my ability to deliver. Her patience is immeasurable and, for that, I am grateful. Thank you to Michael Hawkes and Jessica Morofke for putting up with my too numerous questions! Thank you to Jamie Etherington, Editorial Development Manager, and Dan Allen of the book marketing department, both competent people who make my work look good. Thanks also to Mia Yardley, Natalie Mason, Camille Lowe and the production team at Pindar,

New Zealand, for bringing this book to publication, and the many others who are nameless to me as I write but without whom these books would never come to print; each has his/her stamp on any successes of this book.

My sincere thanks to all of you named, and unnamed, my friends and colleagues along my sometimes broken career path: those who have touched my life in a positive way – and a few, a negative way (for we can learn from the negative to ensure we do better for others).

A final heartfelt statement: any errors, omissions, inaccuracies or deficiencies within these pages are my sole responsibility.

Dedication

I dedicate this book to:

➤ Ella Maisy Cooper (13), a remarkably gifted, gentle-spirited and loving young adult
➤ Megan Louise Feast (10), a considerate, caring, fun-loving and thoughtful child
➤ Daisy Mae Cooper (9), a bright and passionate child, full of heart
➤ Daniel John Charlie Hall (8), a real boy's boy of fun and delight, with a warm, loving and caring nature
➤ Noah Jacob (3), a real sweetheart with good-hearted mischief and fun written in his eyes throughout the day.

Each of you shows love and caring, as it should be, to those around you. How can we resist you – all of you are equal in our hearts and special to us in so many ways. You are all wonderful to Nana and Poppy/Granddad, who are rightly so pleased with all your achievements and successes. May life bring you the joy, pleasure and love you deserve.

CHAPTER 1

Setting the scene

David B Cooper

If I want to know what you're thinking right now, all I have to do is care more about what you're thinking than what I am thinking. . . . As soon as I care more about what you're thinking than what I'm thinking I will give up my thoughts and I will absorb yours, and I will understand.[1]

INTRODUCTION

The difficulties encountered by people who experience mental health–substance use problems are not new. The individual using substances can often encounter annoyance and suspicion when presenting to the mental health professional. Likewise, the person experiencing mental health problems, when presenting to the substance use services, can encounter hostility and hopelessness. 'We cannot do anything for the substance use problem until the mental health problem is dealt with!' The referral to the mental health team is returned: 'We cannot do anything for this person until the substance use problem is dealt with!' Thus, the individual is in the middle of two professional worlds and neither is willing to move, yet both professional worlds are involved in 'caring' for the individual.

For many years, it has been acknowledged that the two parts of the caring system need to work as one. However, this desire has not developed into practice. Over recent years, the impetus has changed; there is now a drive towards meeting the needs of the individual experiencing combined mental health–substance use problems by pooling expertise from both sides. Moreover, there is an international political will to bring about change, often driven forward by a small group of dedicated professionals at practice level.

Some healthcare environments have merely paid lip service – ensuring the correct terminology is included within the policy and procedure documentation, while at the same time doing nothing, or little, to bring about the changes needed at the practice level. Others have grasped the drive forward and have spearheaded developments at local and national level to meet such needs. There now appears to be a concerted international effort to improve the services provided for the individual, and a determination to pool knowledge and expertise. In addition, there is the ability of these professional groups to link into government policy and bring about the political will to support such change. However, this cannot happen overnight.

Major attitudinal changes are needed – not least at management and practice level; one consultant commented that to work together on mental health–substance use problems would be too costly. Furthermore, the consultant believed it would create 'too much work'! Consequently, there is a long way to go – but there *is* a driving force to succeed.

Obtaining in-depth and knowledgeable text is difficult in new areas of change. One needs to be motivated to trawl a broad spectrum of work in order to develop the sound grounding that is needed to build good professional practice. This is a big request of the hard-worked and pressured professional. There are a few excellent mental health–substance use books available. However, this series of six books, of which this is the fifth, is groundbreaking, in that each presents a much-needed text that will introduce the vital steps to the interventions and treatments available for the individual experiencing mental health–substance use concerns and dilemmas.

These books are educational. However, they will make no one an expert! In mental health–substance use, there is a need to initiate and maintain education and training. There are key principles and factors we need to bring out and explore. Some we will use, others we will adapt and others we will reject. Each book is complete. Conversely, each aims to build on the preceding book. However, books **do not** hold all the answers. Nothing does. What is hoped is that the professional will participate in, and collaborate with, each book, progressing through each to the next. Along the way, hopefully, the professional will enhance existing knowledge or develop new concepts to benefit the individual.

The books offer a first step, relevant to the needs of professionals – at practice level or senior service development – in a clear, concise and understandable format. Each book has made full use of boxes, tables, figures, interactive exercises, self-assessment tools and case studies – where appropriate – to examine and demonstrate the effect mental health–substance use can have on the individual, family, carers and society as a whole.

A deliberate attempt has been made to avoid jargon, and where special terminology is used, to offer a clear explanation and understanding. The terminology used is fully explained at the beginning of each book, before the reader commences with the chapters. By placing it there the reader will be able to reference it quickly, if needed. Specific gender is used, as the author feels appropriate. However, unless stated, the use of the male/female gender is interchangeable.

BOOK 5: CARE IN MENTAL HEALTH–SUBSTANCE USE

Case study 1.1

My life was good, a home, family, work. I lived for work because that provided me with the money to keep my family – my responsibility. But things were going wrong, I lost control of my perceived destiny. Ill health took control. Initially, I coped, I had hope, it will get better – no need to adapt – but the system was slow; stepped care meant that I could not get back my usual good health. I had to try this before I could try that – even though I knew 'that' would help me! Then I entered my 'abyss'.

The darkness as I call it took over. It might take days, weeks, months, years, to clear – maybe never – at that time I did not know! 'Eventually you will find a way to cope and accept.' At this stage this was just a myth put about by 'them'. Just something your family and friends told you. Slowly they stepped back unable to cope with my behaviour and actions. I was angry, sad, despairing, unhappy, unreasonable, and obnoxious! I built a brick wall around me. Each meeting with the specialist brought initial hope – then hopelessness. I tried to recreate what I had and cocoon myself in my own safe world. My income dropped – disappeared altogether – but the bills did not! But society and state perceive people like me as scroungers – work dodgers – a burden. In my mind I was begging for money. But my income was not as it was – I needed money to keep things as they were. I created my own empire – borrowed money I could not pay back in the misguided belief that this would bring normality back to my life – and I would then pay my debts. My debtors were after me, my family wanted me to change – but there was no way out or so I believed. I felt ashamed – I hid things – my feelings – my life was a lie – because no one would understand. I sank into a hole; maybe sought thrills. I would buy something that I believed would make me happy, but I didn't need it, and the happiness passed as soon as I bought the expensive 'treat'! Nobody cared – or that is how I felt – I will die – indeed, I wanted to die. I acted in ways I did not understand – and again the shame, the despair – no way out – so what – who cares! Some sort of self-harm, self-gratification – all was doomed, I would get the punishment I deserved for being ill – not like normal hardworking people. I wanted to be punished – needed to be punished – punished for being weak and ill – not normal. At some point I accepted that I needed to change – to adapt – to take control of 'it'. It cannot be in charge of me. I accepted my position in life – the illness – its potential route. Slowly I came out of my abyss. I looked around and saw the damage I had done. I was aware of the destruction – but helpless. I tried to make amends and build bridges with those I had hurt along the way. Some may forgive – others may accept – while others will never forgive or accept. The damage lives alongside my illness. But I saw a light – my own light of acceptance. I accepted the progression of my illness. Of course, many people have helped me along the way – but that goes unacknowledged. I needed to do this for myself. Now I accept the good days – and the bad. I know the damage to myself is progressive – and the damage to others cannot be corrected – but I can only accept my future. Yes, there are down days – black, cold and empty days. But I look for hope. Hang on to the hope – for that is my way forward – my way out. Until the end! Of course, this is my story – my life. We are all different – I suppose we handle things differently. But that is how it was for me – then and now.

The case study above offers an insight into the life journey of the individual experiencing mental health–substance use problems. We do not know how it is for him/her but we listen to the individual's story. The professional's role is to see where the individual is in his/her life. To support and steer that individual to a level of stability that is acceptable to him/her. You may not be able to 'fix', but may be able to encourage acceptance and bring hope – to offer 'care' to the individual.

But what of the person who cares for the carer – the professional – does she/he need care? This book is primarily about caring for the individual and family who come to us for care at a time when their lives are unmanageable alone. However, we must at the same time address the issue of looking after the professional who cares for the individual/family. If we are to provide good-quality care then we need to ensure that the carers themselves (in this case the professionals) are cared for.

It is strange that a 'caring profession', which cares for the ill and troubled, can turn on ill colleagues and apply rules to ensure they return to work quickly. Such as chasing up, without considering that the professional may also need care. We introduce one change after another, increasing the workload of front-line professionals, removing resources and downgrading – shortages are the norm rather than the exception – and yet we do little to support the professionals who are affected.

Change is unsettling and yet we permit rumour to spread about redundancies and demotions without meeting directly to explain what is going on – this is management by 'fear', sometimes bullying – and it is wrong! If communication were effective then it would be possible to bring the professional onside with change; if it were balanced and even-handed it could be achieved quickly and effectively. However, there appears to be a perception that 'they', the front-line professionals, do not need to know until the time is perceived to be right. Working in such a manner causes friction and directly affects the care of the individual and family.

It is imperative that we care effectively and efficiently for the professional at all levels. Robust clinical supervision, supported education and training and inclusion in decision-making are all easy to introduce and have little cost impact. Yet, we fail to consider the needs of the carer persistently, under the illusion that 'they' do not need to be cared for, 'their' job is to care for others. To improve the quality of care for the individual and family this attitude needs to change. But it will take more than a comment in a single chapter to change the philosophy of care for all people including the professional. Surely we are in the business of caring and want to achieve a good standard of care for the individual and family? To be effective in that business we need to care for the carers – so who will be first to bring about this change? Effective communication is the starting point . . .

It costs more to employ a *new* professional than to care for the professional we already have – it is more cost-effective and makes sense . . . so why does it not happen?

The professional's role is to see where the individual is in his/her life, to support and steer that individual to a level of stability that is acceptable to him/her. You may not be able to 'fix', but may be able to encourage acceptance and bring hope. This is also the manager's responsibility to her/his employees. There is no difference in the care that is needed for the individual, family and professional. Nor should we forget that we need to care for the manager's well-being. It is not merely a 'them down to us' process but a two-way interaction of humanness in the face of what can be a very hard – but rewarding – occupation.

As we look at the role of caring in this book and how it can enhance the health and well-being of the individual and family in our care, remember to consider how this caring should be extended and applied to our professional colleagues.

'We should judge ourselves before we judge others.'

For the individual and family it is important that we intervene in a way that is right for the individual – what works for one person may not work for another. Matching the intervention to the person leads to a more effective outcome. Working with the individual in a supportive environment, alongside others experiencing similar problems, should not be overlooked as an effective intervention.

The professional listens to and works alongside the individual as he/she moves towards their goals. Sometimes one way does not work and an alternative is tried – the good professional never gives up on the individual – no one 'deserves it'. The door should always be open – the professional accepting of the individual at whatever point she/he enters our care (*see* Book 1, Chapter 7).

To achieve this, the professional needs an understanding of what is available to aid the individual in achieving his/her own goals: where he/she wants to be and what is acceptable to him/her – not what is acceptable to the professional! To do this we need the basics – then we develop that knowledge into practice and skill.

As mentioned in the Preface, the ability to learn and gain new knowledge is the way forward. As professionals, we must start with knowledge, and from there we can begin to understand. We commence using our new-found skills, and then develop the ability to examine practice, to put concepts together and to make valid judgements.[2] This knowledge is gained through education, training and experience, sometimes enhanced by our own life experiences.

Those we offer care to, and their family members, bring their own knowledge, skills and life experiences, some developed from dealing with ill health. Therefore, mutual understanding and respect is necessary to make interventions and treatment outcome effective.

We need to appreciate and understand the concerns and dilemmas that face the person before she/he comes for advice and treatment. We have to adapt the service to respond to those individual needs. It is important to remember that each person is unique. Yes, there may be similarities in symptoms, and specific needs relevant to sex and age. However, we must accept and acknowledge that each will have variations and specific needs that have to be considered when developing appropriate services, and when interacting with the individual. Moreover, we must be aware of the needs of the family and carers, who have their own specific needs.

To get to this level of skill we need a grounding – a sound knowledge of the theories behind the treatments – how they work, who may benefit, the principles behind the interventions. Practice must be research led and be fluid enough to be updated and modified as knowledge and skills progress. These are the philosophies and ethics – the grounding – from which effective interventions are introduced and developed. This book describes the various models of care available to address the concerns and dilemmas faced by the individual and family. To provide effective care there is a need for a 'starting point' of intervention; then an understanding of the types of interventions that may improve the quality of life for the person and family. To this end, Book 5 provides the basis of best current practice in caring for the individual and family.

Chapter 2 begins the move to developing services by looking at how we access services and how such access can be improved. This chapter seeks to highlight a range of strategies and practices that enhance access to treatment for individuals with diverse mental health–substance use needs.

In Chapter 3, Shona McIntosh looks at improving access to psychological interventions and expresses that '[w]e sometimes have to make the best of what we have. This involves thinking differently.' This chapter outlines ways of improving access to psychological services. It offers a working example within a stepped care pathway. It is hoped this chapter will 'facilitate new ways of thinking about service design and improved access to interventions'.

Alison Sadler, in Chapter 4, offers an insight into the things we need to consider as professionals when we care for the family. The needs and expectations of the family are often forgotten and undermined, especially when we are developing or changing services for the individual, and yet they are key to well-being.

In Chapter 5, Charlotte de Crespigny and Seekar Valadian focus our attention on the needs and expectations when caring for Indigenous peoples – in this case the Indigenous populations of Australia. However, the care, guidance and skills required can and should be applicable to any population, no matter where we live in the world. It is a matter of cultural respect. It should form the basis of any care we offer.

Chapter 6 summarises the evidence for effectively working alongside young people. Ian Wilson explores issues of mental health–substance use and looks at ways of influencing professional attitudes and values towards these individuals, and of enhancing knowledge and skills. Practical ways of engaging distressed young people are proposed and discussed.

In Chapter 7, David Watkins and colleagues encourage readers to consider and reflect on the important role the professional plays when engaging the individual and family. They discuss ways in which the professional can engage and work with families experiencing mental health–substance use problems, and how the professional can use 'self' and their relationships when engaging the individual and family. They also consider how service systems can be used to introduce effective and sustainable change.

In Chapter 8, Brian Rush and Saulo Castel offer an in-depth look at screening and screening tools. The authors focus on evidence-based screening and advocate that screening should be routine for those we care for, be that person an adult, a young or older person or a child.

Mick Adams and Gemma Stacey-Emile address assessment in Chapter 9. This is an in-depth work that looks at the humanistic side of assessment and the cultural considerations needed for effective assessment in an ongoing process throughout the care of the individual and family.

Chapter 10 addresses brief intervention. Karl Robins and David Hingley emphasise how important it is to use a person-centred approach and demonstrates the effectiveness of the approach using solution focused brief therapy. The case study shows how the intervention works and how effective this approach can be.

Chapters 11 and 12 complement each other. Chapter 11 – Integrated motivational interviewing and cognitive behavioural intervention, by Michael Fitzsimmons and Christine Barrowclough– focuses on the Motivational Interventions for Drugs and

Alcohol misuse in Schizophrenia (MIDAS) Trial. The chapter expands on previous descriptions and provides detail with an extended case study. Taking a closer look at the model, the chapter reviews current understanding of interactions between psychosis and substances. Derek Tobin, in Chapter 12, looks at how an integrated treatment philosophy led to the development of a cognitive behavioural integrated treatment (C-BIT) model. The chapter looks at how this treatment manual developed, and how the education and training needs of the professional were met in implementing this approach. A case study is presented to demonstrate how this treatment approach works in practice.

Therapeutic interventions play an important role in the care of the individual. However, we should not forget the role medication has to offer in symptom management. In Chapter 13, Cynthia Geppert and Kenneth Minkoff emphasise the importance of (a) recognising that people experiencing mental health problems may also have substance use problems and (b) being aware of the potential interactions between prescribed medication and these other substances. That does not mean that prescribed medication cannot, or should not, be used and this chapter explores how effective management can be beneficial to the individual. Je Kan Adler-Collins is a Buddhist monk who, in Chapter 14, examines complementary and alternative therapy and its place for the individual experiencing mental health–substance use problems. If we are to successfully offer person-centred care we cannot close the door to any intervention that might be effective for the individual; the individual must have freedom to decide what does and does not work for him/her. This chapter offers a brief look outside the 'comfort circle' at interventions that may be helpful if we are to match need to effective intervention. In light of this the reader is asked to step back, consider who it is we are serving and what that person needs in order to achieve his or her chosen goal. Only through expanding our approach to care can we offer a truly human person-centred approach to care.

Book 5 concludes with Chapter 15, by Peter Athanasos and colleagues looking at the complicated role of pain management. It demonstrates that pain should not be undermanaged just because there is a substance use problem, nor should we assume that a person experiencing substance use problems will misuse prescribed pain management medication. The chapter emphasises that we should not exclude physical problems – that they may coexist with mental health–substance use problems, and are an important part of the assessment and management process. None exists in isolation!

CONCLUSION

We must remember that there is a constant theme throughout in relation to the need for properly funded education and training, for both the professional and individual. Just as important, there is constant reinforcement of why we need to know about mental health–substance use. This book is aimed at the professional, educator, service developer, manager and student, for we all need to be aware of the unique needs of the individual and of interventions available if our practice is to be effective.

I hope that this book is helpful and informative. I hope that readers will feel sufficiently stimulated to further develop their knowledge and skills, having extended and developed this grounding in mental health–substance use. We can build upon our knowledge using the 'To Learn More' sections as a guide to further study and knowledge. As one enters each new area of knowledge, so our understanding improves – of what is needed, and what is not, and of how we can apply this knowledge in practice and service development. With that comes the ability to use an open, non-judgemental and accepting approach to the problems identified by the individual presenting for intervention, treatment, advice or guidance.

Our knowledge and understanding constantly change. The challenge is to remain open and accessible to the knowledge and information that will help each of us provide appropriate therapeutic interventions

➤ at the appropriate level of expertise
➤ at the appropriate time
➤ at the appropriate level of understanding of the individual, and her/his presenting concerns and dilemmas
➤ at the appropriate cost.

We cannot afford to be solid in the belief that all individuals are the same. If this book encourages us to be wise and flexible in practice and the development and provision of services, it has achieved its aim. If it helps us to appreciate some of the problems encountered by the individual, family and carers, it has achieved its aim. We can bring about much-needed change for the individual experiencing mental health–substance use problems.

> 'Respect leads to caring – a quality of impeccability in what we do. Respect and faith nourish each other and give birth to many skilful actions. As we foster the quality of respect in our lives, we can also begin to see the world in a different light. The tone of caring that arises from giving respect can transform how we interact with society. We begin to explore the possibility of service, of taking an active role in seeing what needs doing and lending our energy to those endeavours. Compassion motivates us to act, and wisdom ensures the means are effective.'[3]

REFERENCES

1 Solomon P. Paul Solomon speaks on spiritual roots and the journey to wholeness. *Human Potential Magazine*. 1991; **16**: 28–32.
2 Bloom BS, Hastings T, Madaus G. *Handbook of Formative and Summative Evaluation*. New York, NY: McGraw-Hill Book Company; 1971.
3 Joseph Goldstein. As cited in: Föllmi D, Föllmi O. *Buddhist Offerings 365 Days*. London: Thames & Hudson; 2003.

CHAPTER 2

Accessing services

Kim Moore

REFLECTIVE PRACTICE EXERCISE 2.1

Time: 10 minutes
What is it that makes services and treatment accessible to those who want and
need them?

INTRODUCTION

When an individual seeks or obtains treatment, do we appreciate their circumstances: that their decisions are influenced by personal choice, perceived need,
cultural influence, healthcare provision and financial constraints?[1] In mental
health–substance use, access is complicated by additional difficulties – barriers
that are duplicated and magnified leading to a 'double jeopardy'[2] where individuals
are not viewed as suitable candidates in either substance use or in mental health
treatment programmes[3] and access to treatment is denied. While there is now
recognition of the particular needs presented by the individual experiencing combined mental health–substance use problems, and the development and delivery of
excellent specialist clinical services has improved, there continues to be significant
variation in the provision of services for the individuals needing them.

Health services are currently focused on delivering treatment within significant
financial constraints. However, making treatment accessible remains a priority
and in mental health–substance use this continues to be a steep learning curve.
Developing access pathways, marketing services and making them attractive to
use is a complex task that is the precursor to engaging in treatment. The strategic
direction any organisation takes to increase accessibility needs to account for a
range of options offered at different levels of intensity and sophistication, with
consideration given to working as independent specialist services or in cooperative
partnerships. Learning from the experience of the individual, families, colleagues,
public sector and private enterprise has prompted strategic change in the delivery
of treatment and in the access pathways used by individuals experiencing mental
health–substance use problems. This chapter seeks to highlight a range of strategies

and practices that are currently working to enhance access to treatment for individuals with diverse mental health–substance use needs.

Increasing access to mental health–substance use treatment requires a broad-spectrum approach incorporating

➤ primary care
➤ secondary care
➤ self-help
➤ strategic planning

. . . each having its central function but also intrinsically interlinked (*see* Figure 2.1).

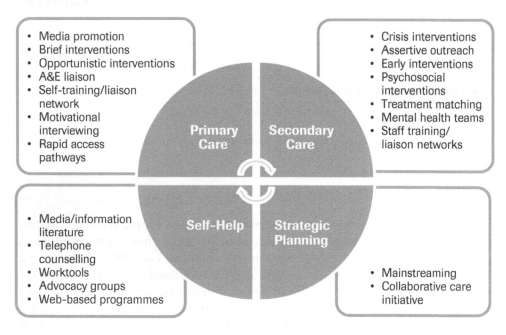

- Media promotion
- Brief interventions
- Opportunistic interventions
- A&E liaison
- Self-training/liaison network
- Motivational interviewing
- Rapid access pathways

Primary Care

Secondary Care

- Crisis interventions
- Assertive outreach
- Early interventions
- Psychosocial interventions
- Treatment matching
- Mental health teams
- Staff training/ liaison networks

- Media/information literature
- Telephone counselling
- Worktools
- Advocacy groups
- Web-based programmes

Self-Help

Strategic Planning

- Mainstreaming
- Collaborative care initiative

FIGURE 2.1 Increasing access to mental health–substance use treatment

USING MEDIA STRATEGIES

One of the common themes in literature crossing healthcare boundaries is how to make services attractive and accessible to those who need them. Health promotion and treatment provision are commodities that can be sold; effective marketing strategies promote initiation of help seeking and direct the individual towards engaging in effective treatment packages. Health promotion teams have been at the forefront of developing and delivering strategies to influence public opinion on sensitive health issues. Embedded within these messages is factual information with directions on where and how to access treatment, resulting in programmes that significantly influence the health behaviour of the targeted population.[4] Health promotion in psychiatry and substance use has focused on reducing the stigma of both health issues, and promoting access to services through multiple treatment entry points. Designing or applying strategies that increase access to mental health–substance use treatment needs to incorporate knowledge learned through promoting sensitive health issues, and use modern marketing strategies to convey the information to individuals needing the service.

Most health organisations working in the public sector focus their strategies on the person in a 'needs-led' service. Access to services is promoted by understanding need and developing services to meet those needs. Marketing strategies are not just about selling a service or disseminating information; healthcare marketing involves establishing a core strategy message with mechanisms to plan and deliver that service. The practicalities of delivering accessible healthcare involve marketing principles that

➤ embrace and use available technology
➤ meet the expressed needs of the individual
➤ promote services to the general public in standardised and innovative ways
➤ are supported by physically accessible buildings
➤ ensure excellent individualised care.

Organisational marketing strategies work to build the reputation of a service, making it attractive to the user and making it stand out from its competitors. The use of marketing strategies is equally relevant in mental health–substance use services.

With mental health–substance use, the fundamental differences in treatment philosophy continue to affect the accessibility of treatment, making the marketing of these services to the public and other professional groups confusing, potentially creating barriers. On a professional level, individuals experiencing mental health–substance use problems are often described as a 'hard-to-reach' treatment group.[5,6] Increasing acceptability and accessibility requires a multilayered approach by professionals, organisations and services; first by addressing their own issues in working with mental health–substance use problems; second, by understanding how and why an individual seeks help. Services are more able to match the treatment access points by using combinations of

➤ strategic change
➤ collaborative and mainstreamed treatment programmes
➤ assertive outreach
➤ stepped care
➤ managed-care programmes
➤ training initiatives that are supported by information technology–based marketing strategies.

CARE AND THE ENVIRONMENT

The starting point for improving access is within individual organisations and teams. It depends on the desire, ability and inclusion of services to work with individuals in such a way that mental health–substance use problems are viewed and treated concurrently as primary problems.[7] Inclusive and accessible services for mental health–substance use are determined by professionals who have a positive attitude towards these issues, and organisations that work to address changing attitudes through education.[8,9] In combination with marketing and education strategies, individualised care delivery improves the processes individuals can use to seek help.[10] Quality care links high-quality information that is easily used and portable with prompt attention and minimum waiting, to enable and support individualised choice.[11] Marketing and individualised care strategies from private enterprise provide examples of promoting services and accessing products by influencing social opinion – 'In our factory, we make lipstick', 'In our advertising, we sell hope.'[12] Looking outside of the health system to private enterprise can provide organisations and professionals with new ideas for improving access to mental health–substance use services.

The final element to consider, in making services accessible to individuals experiencing mental health–substance use problems, is more tangible: the environmental aspects of the building including disabled and pram access. Comfortable furniture and the small touches in decor are important in improving the quality of the experience when accessing services.[13] Professionalism in combination with promotional strategies that provide a menu or pathway into different programmes make services more accessible. We all appreciate working within open, friendly settings and are more likely to use a service that is inviting and attractive, with easy telephone access to real people and where expectations of being valued as an individual are met. Services that develop and market treatment programmes for mental health–substance use that also offer good individualised care are more likely to not only attract the individual but also increase the likelihood that individuals will initiate and remain in treatment.

PROMOTING HEALTH SEEKING IN PRACTICE

What provokes a person to seek help is the sense that something is wrong. Research has demonstrated that initial access to treatment is often through peer networks, advice from general practitioners and accessing Internet information.[13,14] As information technology crosses most cultural and social boundaries it represents a powerful tool that is being used not only to signpost treatment but also to provide treatment.[15]

The growing market of Internet health-promotion sites, chat rooms, telephone counselling, virtual web groups, interactive DVDs and text messaging is testament to the change in accessible treatment. While most of these programmes are aimed at individuals motivated towards self-help with psychological distress, anxiety, depression[16] and substance use problems,[17] they are less developed for mental health–substance use problems. Information technology resources are often easier to access at times and places suitable to the individual; the appeal of these programmes is 'real-time' accessibility, anonymity and entertainment value.[18,19] Innovative interactive programmes like virtual reality and gaming programmes offer immediate access to health education for professionals and for the general public. There are several significant drawbacks to web-based programmes – the emergence of 'extreme communities',[18] addiction to the Internet,[20] the unreliability of information, the accessibility and faith in the technology being the most noted.

When you raise awareness of a health issue, it is important to have a range of strategies to meet that need. Maximising the use of media technology provides rapid access to relevant treatment information and pathways to other treatment modalities. The first access point is web information that is clear, easy to use and informative[21] – being able to print promotional and educational literature creates instant access. Some individuals experiencing mental health–substance use problems are motivated to access self-help treatment. By combining self-help with remote-access strategies, workbooks, informational DVDs, CDs, audio books and telephone counselling we can create more choices for treatment access. Multimedia strategies have an important place for increasing accessibility. However, in order to be effective they need to be cost-effective, use clear and simple language, be informative and provide signposts for further help seeking. Enhancing access to mental health–substance use services for motivated individuals includes being able to offer a range of treatment choices that can be undertaken alone, or can be combined with remote guidance or signposting to other access options.

PROMOTING ACCESS IN COMPLEX CASES

Thus far, the focus for creating and enhancing access to mental health–substance use services has centred on
➤ building business frameworks that are attractive to the individual
➤ providing immediate and remote access, with clear information/signposting
➤ self-help treatments.

Using business strategies with individuals who are more reluctant or avoidant of traditional services remains important. However, increased clinical interactions delivered at varying levels of intensity and flexibility work to enhance treatment access by providing a wider range of options.[22] Accessing treatment is multilayered; we should assume that there have been multiple attempts and failures in accessing treatment through many avenues and sources.[23] We know that individuals experiencing mental health–substance use problems can and do seek access to treatment through
➤ accident and emergency departments
➤ general practitioners
➤ healthy-living centres
➤ pharmacists

. . . often with less reluctance than accessing secondary treatment services, so what is it that makes these services more accessible?

REFLECTIVE PRACTICE EXERCISE 2.2

Time: 10 minutes
Reflect on what could be done – by you and your organisation – to make services more accessible. Make a list of your perceptions.

For many years, primary care services provided mental health–substance use treatment through episodes of unplanned, ad hoc or crisis care. While this relationship has not always been harmonious, there is a general understanding that these are the services to be used when needing health information, care and professional help outside of 'standard office hours'. Maximising accessible treatment of mental health–substance use depends on learning from each other, exchanging knowledge, working together and incorporating opportunistic interventions in shared vision of treatment, at all levels of healthcare. Shifting mainstream models towards collaborative care networks, where primary care is at the heart of service accessibility and delivery of treatment,[24] recognises the significant contribution made by these services. Primary care pathways aimed at accessing mental health–substance use treatment show promise for engaging diverse cultural groups in symptom recognition and treatment initiation (*see* Chapters 5 and 9; Book 4, Chapters 4 and 5).[25,26] Ultimately, the primary care service – the general practitioner in particular – undertakes many roles, often being initiator, facilitator and ongoing care provider.

Making mental health–substance use services accessible has become the focus for developing formalised collaborative care pathways. Systemic collaborative care programmes are important.[27] However, the human factor is also required to deliver the promise that collaboration offers. If we believe that individuals with severe and complex mental health–substance use problems are disenfranchised, avoidant or 'hard to reach'[3] – that we have nothing to offer – then professional beliefs become the barrier to treatment. In the past it was not uncommon for motivated individuals to seek treatment for one element of their perceived problems at the agency where they perceive their needs would be met, only to be turned away as 'unsuitable'; access to treatment was denied. Most services have moved on from this position with systemic policy statements such as the 'no wrong door' and mainstreaming initiatives.[28,29] However, the initial experience of help-seeking individuals has created a negative reputation for services. Learning to change preconceived notions is the business of the professional and agencies working with mental health–substance use problems.

Change can be difficult for all involved. While there is a greater confidence for working with mental health–substance use problems, the severe and highly complex cases continue to challenge personal, professional and service beliefs. Changing public perception, professional practice and service structures are all elements that increase accessibility. Evidence suggests that when these are combined with rapid and flexible treatment options there is an increase in service satisfaction, improvement in service reputation and an increase in access to treatment.[30,31] The individuals that all services find the most difficult to attract are those with severe cognitive impairment. From the individual's perspective, agencies are frustrating and intimidating.[32]

There is a wealth of knowledge on the treatment of serious mental illness that is applicable to mental health–substance use – in particular, the use of early and integrated psychosocial treatment.[33] The philosophy and practice of integrated teams such as assertive outreach, early interventions and liaison services increases the accessibility of services by taking the service to the person, in her/his own environment. Unlike mental health services, there has been no consistent investment in developing integrated mental health–substance use practices, effectively creating a health lottery. Many have argued that specialist mental health–substance use teams, while valuable, are an ineffective use of resources, with finite limitations on the number of individuals able to access treatment at any given time. Maximising access to services for the complex individual experiencing mental health–substance use problems incorporates all the techniques used for motivated individuals, and enhances access by taking the service to the individual as a standard practice.[34-36]

In the most complex of cases, access to treatment is more often coercive. Of the many parallels among mental health, substance use problems and criminal justice systems, the use of coercive strategies is one of the most controversial, and arguably most overused, means of expediting access to treatment. While organisations are working to reduce coercive practices, these strategies are often subtle and highly prevalent in ensuring access in all treatment services.[37] There are occasions when involuntary mental health admission needs to be used in mental health–substance use practice. This is based solely on the mental health presentation. There are many different methods of persuasion or leverage used to promote treatment access; examples of social and financial rewards for individuals entering treatment can be found throughout the literature.[38] In some countries the offer of free treatment or cash payment to attend is the incentive used to promote access to treatment. There is a fine line between using coercion, leverage and behavioural rewards and describing these as motivational enhancement techniques.[37]

SYSTEMIC CHANGE TO PROMOTE ACCESS

Innovations in promotion and delivery of mental health–substance use services lead to systemic changes within the wider national health agenda. The most recognised of these strategies are mainstreaming and collaborative care. Based on the principle that mental health–substance use problems are expected, all services have a mandated responsibility to provide access to treatment across treatment sectors. Many obstacles to accessing treatment can be overcome by designing complementary and seamless pathways that are responsive to needs and are delivered in familiar surroundings. The expectation of mainstream working or collaborative care by multiple providers means that services work to their organisational strengths. Moreover, there is mutual support and learning from one another that impact across all professionals providing treatment access. Systems alone cannot support increasing accessibility of services for mental health–substance use problems. However, they make a significant impact on reducing professional and social barriers to treatment. Systemic change is directly influenced by professionals who advocate on behalf of the individual. This brings expressions of hope, optimism and a positive outlook,[39] and a commitment to change and growth.

CONCLUSION

Health is a business commodity: good individualised care, multimedia strategies and quality treatment packages are all components of providing access to treatment. Mental health–substance use is no exception to this. In business, delivery of financially competitive and quality services is the goal. Developing access pathways requires understanding of the needs of the local community, and service position within this community. There is much to be learned within and outside the healthcare system. Innovative changes in the delivery of mental health–substance use services can make them more accessible and acceptable to the wider public. Using market strategies to enhance access to services can be limited or innovative. How difficult or easy this is depends on us and how we choose to make them.

Access to services is not a simple or linear pathway; individuals experiencing mental health–substance use problems can and do enter into many services at different times for different needs. Developing formal cooperative pathways along a continuum of healthcare providers increases the number of professionals able to offer access to a diversified range of treatment. Increasing individual choice enables earlier and faster access to treatment. It requires professional attitudes towards mental health–substance use problems that are supportive and inclusive – that working with mental health–substance use problems is the norm. Personal and professional qualities including knowledge, hope, understanding, persistence and conviction can and do make a difference to individuals accessing services within local systems, and in provoking and promoting change in others.

There are many levels that single organisations or collaborations among multiple agencies can change to increase accessibility; for example, by making services attractive, by encouraging staff to regard mental health–substance use needs as expected issues and by improving the reputation of the service identity. Many organisations continue to work on reducing treatment barriers within and across treatment systems. This ongoing task continues to evolve. The application of combined strategies improves access to treatment, and the human factor makes it happen. Improving accessibility to mental health–substance use services is a shared responsibility. It is not insurmountable. Organisations and individuals can travel this path alone, or they can work together to promote social and political change on issues that enhance treatment access.

REFERENCES

1 Rickwood D, Deane FP, Wilson CJ, *et al.* Young people's help-seeking for mental health problems. *Medical Journal of Australia.* 2005; **187**: S35–9. Available at: www.mja.com.au (accessed 20 September 2010).

2 Lehman A, Dixon L. *Double Jeopardy: chronic mental illness and substance use disorder.* 1st ed. New Jersey: Hardwood Academic Publishers; 1995.

3 Koekkoek B, Meijel B, Hutschemaekers G. 'Difficult patients' in mental health care: a review. *Psychiatric Services.* 2006; **57**: 795–802.

4 Vanheusden K, van der Ende J, Mulder C, *et al.* Beliefs about mental health problems and help-seeking behaviour in Dutch young adults. *Social Psychiatry and Psychiatric Epidemiology.* 2009; **44**: 239–46.

5 Brackertz N, Zwart I, Meredyth D, *et al. Community Consultation and the 'Hard to Reach': concepts and practice in Victorian local government.* Victoria, Australia: Institute for Social Research, Swinburne University of Technology; 2005.

6 The Scottish Government. *Working with hard to reach young people: a practical guide.* Available at: www.scotland.gov.uk/Publications/2007/12/06145646/0 (accessed 2 March 2011).

7 Cline A, Minkoff K. *Changing the World: welcoming, accessible recovery-orientated culturally fluent comprehensive, continuous, integrated systems of care for individuals and families with psychiatric and substance use disorders.* 2003. Available at: www.isc.idaho.gov/dcourt/Integration%20of%20Treatment%20Minkoff.pdf (accessed 6 February 2011).

8 Hughes E, Wanigaratne S, Gournay K, *et al.* Training in dual diagnosis interventions (the COMO study): randomised controlled trial. *BMC Psychiatry.* 2008; **8**: 12. Available at: www.biomedcentral.com/bmcpsychiatry/ (accessed 20 September 2010 – free registration required to access the documents).

9 Renner J. How to train residents to identify and treat dual diagnosis. *Society of Biological Psychiatry*. 2004; **56**: 810–16.

10 Smith T. E, Burgos J, Dexter V, *et al*. Best practice: best practices for improving engagement of clients in clinic care. *Psychiatric Services*. 2010; **61**: 343–5.

11 *Start up Briefing: how to involve your whole team in customer care*. London: BHP Information Solutions; 2009. ISSN 1469–0470. Available at: www.icaew.com/enterprise/db/pdf/11cuscar. pdf (accessed 4 October 2010).

12 Revlon. Available at: www.revloninc.com (accessed 20 September 2010).

13 Brems J, Brennan E, Epperson K, *et al*. *More Than a Waiting Room*. 2009. Available at: http:// neuroanthropology.net/2009/01/25/more-than-a-waiting-room/ (accessed 20 September 2010).

14 heretohelp. Available at: www.heretohelp.bc.ca (accessed 20 September 2010).

15 Gray N, Klein J, Noyce P, *et al*. Health information-seeking behaviour in adolescence: the place of the internet. *Social Science and Medicine*. 2005; **60**: 1467–78.

16 Bell V. Online information, extreme communities and Internet therapy: is the Internet good for our mental health? *Journal of Mental Health*. 2007; **16**: 445–57.

17 *Using Self-Help Techniques to Addiction Free*. Available at: www.beatingaddictions.co.uk (accessed 20 September 2010).

18 Sullivan C, Morrison M, Lee K, editors. *The RORRT: young people using the web to promote positive mental health*. 6th National Rural Health Conference, 2001. ACT: Australia.

19 *A Virtual Gaming World to Help Young People Get through Tough Times*. Inspire Foundation; 2007. Available at: http://roc.reachout.com.au/flash/index.html (accessed 20 September 2010).

20 *Internet Addiction Disorder*. Available at www.minddisorders.com (accessed 20 September 2010).

21 Kalk N, Pothier D. Patient information on schizophrenia on the Internet. *Psychiatric Bulletin*. 2008; **32**: 409–11.

22 Chen S, Barnett P, Sempel J, *et al*. Outcomes and costs of matching the intensity of dual-diagnosis treatment to patients' symptom severity. *Journal of Substance Abuse Treatment*. 2006; **31**: 95–105.

23 Ghanizadeh A, Arkan N, Mohammadi M, *et al*. Frequency of and barriers to utilization of mental health services in an Iranian population. *Eastern Mediterranean Health Journal*. 2008; **14**: 438–46. Available at: www.emro.who.int/publications/emhj/1402/article23.htm (accessed 20 September 2010).

24 Bonsack C, Adam L, Haefliger T, *et al*. Difficult-to-engage patients: a specific target for time-limited assertive outreach in a Swiss setting. *Canadian Journal of Psychiatry*. 2005; **50**: 845–50.

25 Merrritt-Davis O, Keshaven M. Pathways to care for African Americans with early psychosis. *Psychiatric Services*. 2006; **57**: 1043–4.

26 Oliver M, Pearson N, Coe N, *et al*. Help-seeking behaviour in men and women with common mental health problems: cross-sectional study. *British Journal of Psychiatry*. 2005; **186**: 297–301.

27 Gournay K, Sandford T, Johnson S, *et al*. Dual diagnosis of severe mental health problems and substance abuse/dependence: a major priority for mental health nursing. *Journal of Psychiatric and Mental Health Nursing*. 1997; **4**: 89–95.

28 Webster C, Longhi D, Kohlenberg L. *No Wrong Door: designs of integrated, client centered service plans for persons and families with multiple needs*. Washington, DC: Washington

State Department of Social and Health Services; 2001. Available at: www.dshs.wa.gov/pdf/ms/rda/research/11/99.pdf (accessed 20 September 2010).

29 Morley A. *Mainstreaming Mental Health: an introduction for counsellors*. London: Local Government Information Centre; 2005.

30 Bauer M, McBride L, Shea N, *et al*. Impact of easy-access VA clinic-based program for patients with bipolar disorder. *Psychiatric Services*. 1997; **48**: 491–6.

31 Felker B, Barnes R, Greenberg D, *et al*. Preliminary outcomes from an integrated mental health primary care team. *Psychiatric Services*. 2004; **55**: 442–4.

32 Scott J, Dixon L. Community-based treatment for severe mental illness: what are the benefits and costs? *Medscape Psychiatry & Mental Health eJournal* 1997; **2**(5). Available at: www.medscape.com/viewarticle/430885_3 (accessed 20 September 2010).

33 Mueser KT, Bond GR, Drake RE. Community-based treatment of schizophrenia and other severe mental disorders: treatment outcomes. *Medscape General Medicine*. 2001; **3** [formerly published in *Medscape Psychiatry & Mental Health eJournal* 2001; **6**]. Available at: www.medscape.com/viewarticle/430529 (accessed 20 September 2010).

34 Phillips S, Burns B, Edgar E, *et al*. Moving assertive community treatment into standard practice. *Psychiatric Services*. 2001; **52**: 771–9.

35 Timko C, Sempel J. Short-term outcomes of matching dual diagnosis patients' symptom severity to treatment intensity. *Journal of Substance Abuse Treatment*. 2004; **26**: 209–18.

36 Craven MA, Bland R. *Better Practices in Collaborative Mental Health Care: an analysis of the evidence base*. Canadian Collaborative Mental Health Initiative. 2006. Available at: www.ccmhi.ca/en/products/documents/04_BestPractices_EN.pdf (accessed 20 September 2010).

37 Ellila H, Saarikoski M. Coercive treatment is a challenge for psychiatric nursing in Europe. *International Journal of Psychiatric Nursing Research*. 2004; **10**: 1164–7.

38 Szmukler G, Appelbaum P. Treatment pressures, leverage, coercion and compulsion in mental health care. *Journal of Mental Health*. 2008; **17**: 233–44.

39 Minkoff K. *Behavioral Health Recovery Management Service Planning Guidelines: co-occurring psychiatric and substance disorders*. Illinois: Illinois Department of Human Services Office of Alcoholism and Substance Abuse; 2001.

TO LEARN MORE

- On the Internet or in a health resource library find and read the article by Oliver, *et al.* (2005). Help-seeking behaviour in men and women with common mental health problems: cross-sectional study. *British Journal of Psychiatry*. 2005; **186**: 297–301. This article can also be found at http://bjp.rcpsych.org/cgi/content/full/bjprcpsych;186/4/297 (accessed 23 January 2011). What can you learn from this study that may help promote access to treatment in your service?

- Complete a Google search on self-help for dual diagnosis issues. Based on what you found, what do you consider to be the benefits and drawbacks of this method of seeking information and help?

- Go to the Progress website www.dualdiagnosis.co.uk/DrugAlcoMental.ink and read the story on Jason (accessed 23 January 2011). Reflecting on what you have just seen, list the positive and negative aspects of this as a resource and how it could be used in practice.

- Consider your place of work – what consumer care practices do you have in place that makes your service attractive and accessible to service users?

CHAPTER 3

Improving access to psychological interventions

Shona McIntosh

> 'It's not just what you're born with,
> It's what you choose to bear
> It's not how large your share is,
> But how much you can share
> Oh it's not the fights you dream of
> But those you really fought
> It's not just what you're given
> But what you do with what you've got'[1]

REFLECTIVE PRACTICE EXERCISE 3.1

Time: 15 minutes
You are in the middle of a desert, have 5000 people to feed, and have only five loaves and two fish. The nearest supermarket is a week's walk away; it doesn't do online deliveries and you have got only £20 anyway. You are anxious and feel out of control of the situation. What do you do?

INTRODUCTION

According to the source text of this problem a miracle was performed and all were fed, with baskets of leftovers for future meals.[2] If you do not believe in miracles, or if you look more closely at the texts, it might become evident that a certain amount of emergence and sharing of other skills and resources had taken place among the 5000. Someone may have asked if anyone else had any food. Others may have immediately let it be known that they had food and would share their provisions. A few people may have needed some degree of persuasion and influencing by those with skills in such matters to see the long-term benefits to themselves and others. Those with good foresight may have brought extra food. Others may have had the ability to prepare food so that a little went a long way. A few may not have been as hungry as others. People may have eaten only what they needed rather than engaged in gluttony. Some would have stood back to let others eat. Things were sorted out.

A combination of a range of human behaviour, complexity theory[3-5] and a 'wicked' rather than 'tame'[6] approach may have saved the day.

In the world of substance use it is often a much larger crowd (people with complex problems, their families and those who provide care and services) who need sustenance (access to psychological interventions and therapies) and are challenged by poor or ineffective planning and apparently limited resources and skills in a barren place.

No miracles are foreseen but nor are they ruled out.

CHAPTER AIMS

We sometimes have to make the best of what we have. This involves thinking differently. This chapter aims to:

➤ briefly outline some of the current drivers for improving access to psychological services

➤ give a working example of a consultancy model within a stepped care pathway to improve access to psychological services

➤ suggest further reading to facilitate new ways of thinking about service design and improved access to interventions

➤ highlight some of the learning points in designing and implementing the pathway; that is, what to think about in order to get a service delivered

➤ give suggestions for further learning and promote thinking about other ways to improve access to psychological interventions in future.

WHY DO WE NEED TO IMPROVE ACCESS TO PSYCHOLOGICAL INTERVENTIONS?

Given that you are reading this chapter, it could be assumed that most of you are more interested in *how* to increase access to psychological interventions rather than whether or not there is value in doing so. For those of you who are not quite sure and like detail, this chapter includes a 'To Learn More' section and suggested reading and briefly outlines some of the current drivers to increasing access to psychological interventions.

➤ There is clear evidence for the effectiveness and need for psychological and psychosocial interventions for people with **complex psychological problems and substance use problems across the lifespan**.[7-14] Changes in behaviour and thinking result from evidence-based psychological interventions. Individuals, families, and communities benefit.

➤ There is recognition that access to and availability of psychosocial interventions is currently limited.[15-17] Commitments have been made by the UK Department of Health (DOH) and Governments of the Devolved Nations to increase access to psychosocial interventions.[18-20] Many of these documents – in particular, the Scottish Government's *Essential Care*[10] – highlight the need for substance use professionals to be skilled in the delivery of psychological interventions and in managing disclosure of abuse and trauma.

A STORY OF PSYCHOLOGICAL STEPPED CARE AND CONSULTANCY

The author's role was to set up and improve access to psychological services for substance use problems for three health boards within a managed care network in the east central belt of Scotland. The population of the boards was approximately 1.2 million with a mix of urban, remote and rural communities. The service was to include partners from commissioners, health, social work and voluntary agencies.

There was one loaf and very few fish. Thus, the author was unable to, and had only the occasional desire to, work miracles. A plan was needed!

READING SUGGESTIONS 3.1

The Changing World and Adaptive Leadership

Before reading on, and to help you with your thinking while reading this chapter, you may wish to look at some of the work being done in the fields of leadership and organisational change. Professor Eddie Obeng[5,21-23] has had a considerable impact on the author's thinking in trying to develop services. Obeng's energetic, non-linear and creative thinking around leading and managing projects and change stimulates new ways of approaching challenges. Obeng's primary thesis is that we are now all living in a world where the pace of change (just think technology alone!) has exceeded the pace at which we can learn. We cannot carry on doing the same as we always did and hope this will meet people's needs. When developing services that allow for improved access, we have to do things differently. We have to challenge and change the way we think and relate to those people we are trying to influence. The 'Adaptive Leadership' model developed by Professor Ronald Heifetz,[24] Marty Linsky and colleagues,[25,26] is very helpful in diagnosing, negotiating and meeting the challenges we face in designing and delivering services in a complex and fast-changing world.

MODEL SERVICE PROVISION AND BEST PRACTICE

A scoping exercise was carried out to ascertain priorities for each health board and the stakeholders within each board. In accordance with British Psychological Society (BPS) and UK DOH guidelines[27] a stepped care model of service provision was designed. The model provides the following.

➤ Clinical governance for psychological stepped care, and consultancy to promote engagement of people using the service.
➤ A means of establishing psychological need. A three-level approach has been adopted to quantify the types of psychological skills and interventions required at each level (adapted from Mowbray[28]):
  — Basic psychotherapeutic skills and interventions including the ability to establish rapport, build collaborative relationships and provide supportive counselling. Harm reduction and psycho-education (including use of virtual self-help websites) also come into this category.
  — Skills encompass manualised or protocol-driven psychological approaches such as cognitive behavioural therapy, motivational interviewing and

behaviour modification (*see* Chapters 11 and 12; Book 4, Chapters 7 and 10).

— Skills are specialised, individually tailored approaches, based upon complex psychological formulations that draw on multiple theoretical models.

➤ Consultation clinics[29] that are adapted to include the possibility of the clinical psychologist or accredited therapist joining sessions with key workers, social workers, psychiatrists and so forth to meet with people directly. This makes best use of – and can support – other professionals' psychological skills, and enhances and encourages conscious competence in their service delivery. If, in future, more complex psychological interventions are required, the attendance rate at psychology clinics is usually significantly increased (80% attendance in one board piloting the model).

➤ Clinical supervision for partners. A first evaluation using the Manchester Clinical Supervision Scale[30] has been very positive.

THE PATHWAY

Figure 3.1[31] shows a person's journey through the care pathway. Eligibility criteria for entry to the pathway are twofold.

1 Step one: all partners within the managed care network can request consultancy, clinical supervision or training in relation to psychological aspects of substance use at any tier or level of psychological intervention. Consultation is available to professionals working alongside people who may not be stable in their substance use or do not require to be referred for more comprehensive assessment for psychological interventions to meet their needs.

2 Step two: people with a current history of substance use problems **and** con-current complex psychological problems may be referred for assessment and treatment with clinical psychologist and/or accredited therapist if:

— there are behavioural indicators demonstrating that a person's substance misuse is stable

— the person has consented to or requested psychological assessment or treatment

— the person is engaged with a partner agency and is under medical supervision.

Examples of complex psychological problems include trauma, sexual abuse and post-traumatic stress disorder, anxiety and mood problems, self-harm, chronic pain, functional illness, long-standing comorbidity and neuropsychological impairment.

The service is aimed at people experiencing mental health–substance use problems. The primary problem should not solely be caused by the substance use. Possible indicators for primary psychological problems would be:

➤ pre-existing mental health problems

➤ psychological problems over and above what would be expected as a result of substance use

➤ psychological problems that are hampering a person's treatment progress with the substance use issue – for example, cognitive impairment.

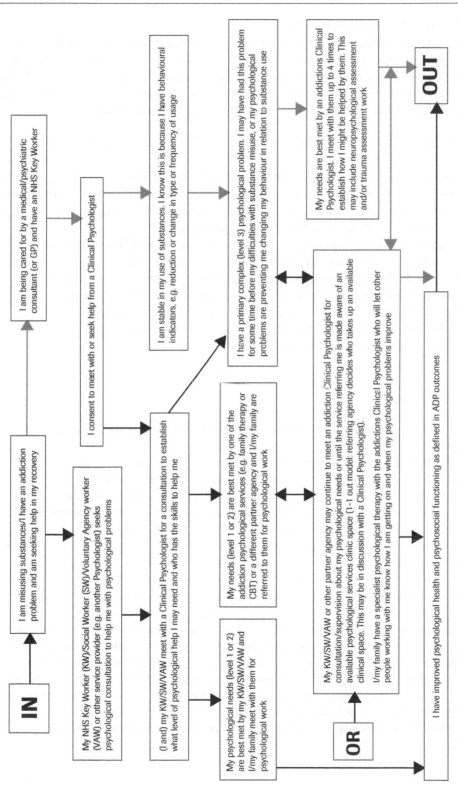

FIGURE 3.1 A person's journey through the care pathway[31]

ONE-IN-ONE-OUT CLINICS

There are specified, limited numbers of direct contact clinics available for post-assessment direct psychological (level 2 and 3) work. When a person is discharged and a space becomes available in clinics referring and consulting agencies (often in consultation with psychology staff) decide who takes up the next clinic space. Consultation with the psychology staff can take place at any time.

HAS THE MODEL WORKED? HAS THERE BEEN AN IMPROVEMENT IN ACCESS TO PSYCHOLOGICAL INTERVENTIONS?

No miracle has occurred but within the first two years of service development the consultancy and supervision model has allowed more people experiencing mental health–substance use problems or other complex needs to access psychological interventions than a conventional clinic-based model.

Applications for funding of posts, within the model described, for clinical psychologists and accredited therapists were successful with some variation across health boards. This was in part due to supportive and visionary colleagues, leadership, a shared set of objectives and good influencing and engagement skills. Due respect has been paid to the need for infrastructure and administration. The number of available loaves and fish has now increased significantly.

Two brief case examples are outlined below.

Case study 3.1: Andrea

A person experiencing substance use problems, trauma and cognitive impairment

Andrea was homeless and unstable in her use of heroin and alcohol. She had been the recent victim of several physical and sexual assaults. Andrea had a child she rarely saw who lived with the child's father. Andrea had been working with a substance use nurse but continually relapsed. The nurse was very concerned about Andrea's vulnerability and sought consultation to help Andrea in her recovery. This led to a psychological assessment that identified a previously undocumented learning disability. Further neuropsychological assessment identified specific cognitive impairments. The clinical psychologist, nurse and consultant psychiatrist were subsequently able to arrange a case conference to look at how different partners might be able to meet Andrea's psychosocial needs. This included adapting materials to accommodate cognitive impairments (using pictorial communication aids and memory aids) and enable better communication with Andrea. This was done in the relapse prevention work and discussions about keeping safe and reducing vulnerability. Andrea went on to have input from a specialist learning-disability nurse, help in finding accommodation and social work involvement to enable her child to have contact with her. Andrea reported no further sexual or physical assaults, and her use of heroin stopped and alcohol use decreased.

Several other people with acquired brain injuries and neuropsychological impairments have been identified and voluntary agency counsellors have been trained in tailoring their counselling interventions to take account of impairments. Examples of this would be teaching the individual to use prospective memory aids (e.g. mobile phone reminders) to enable them to attend appointments, or providing structure and memory aids by means of written résumés of key points in sessions.

Case study 3.2: Tina

A fifteen-year-old with substance use issues living in Looked After Care
Tina came from a family where both her parents used either alcohol or heroin. Most of her life her father had been in prison for selling drugs. Tina had, for the most part, been brought up by her grandmother, who was now saying Tina could no longer live with her due to her behaviour. Tina had been caught shoplifting and was due in front of the Children's Panel for this and several charges of misuse of substances, primarily heroin and benzodiazepine. Tina was known to have been having unprotected sex with a number of older men and there were serious concerns about her behaviour and safety. A member of the Looked After Care (LAC) team brought Tina to supervision with a clinical psychologist. The psychologist later met with Tina during one of the LAC team member sessions and Tina agreed to a further meeting. Further sessions led to Tina, her mother and grandmother agreeing to family therapy with the substance use psychology service family therapist, as part of Tina's recovery.

KEY LEARNING POINTS

➤ In attempting to improve access to services, leadership and skills in leadership are essential. Doing something differently can be viewed or experienced as threatening. The care pathway described (*see* Figure 3.1[31]) relies heavily on best use of the psychological skill mix provided by partners and accredited therapists with clinical governance from clinical psychology. The engagement of partner agencies and stakeholders is vital. Clear goals and limitations need to be agreed before a service-level agreement is made.

➤ Beware of silo thinking and tribal behaviours, which sometimes emerge as survival behaviours in response to perceived threat or change – for example, 'It's always worked this way before . . .', 'We've already tried that . . .', 'What you're suggesting will dumb down interventions . . .', or 'I want my bit to be the best . . .'. You will need to address the political and systemic issues before a service can be delivered. For example, there may be competition between partners for funding for services. You will need at least to be aware of, and preferably find ways of dealing with, such 'elephants'[32] in your discussions or your best efforts may be blocked. While there is a growing emphasis on cross-partner working, old habits die hard and influencing skills are essential. Obeng and Gillet's thinking is useful here[23] as is that of Patterson and colleagues.[33]

➤ Bear in mind that it takes time for people to think differently about service delivery and build this awareness into your plan.

➤ Not all partners speak the same language. There can be wide variation in the skill mix and governance of the UK's National Health Service (NHS), Social Services and the voluntary sector. It is helpful to check that both you and the partner really understand each other. Misconceptions are a frequent cause of poor or dysfunctional engagement. A good example of this is clarity and understanding of what the end product (service) will be. In simple terms, the partner may have a vision of a Michelin-starred meal arriving and will be really upset and disillusioned when presented with a (albeit nutritious) cheese sandwich. You need to be clear how increased access will work for partners.

➤ 'People skills' in engagement and relationships are paramount. This is especially important when you need other people to act on your behalf and, for example, influence those who hold the money for service developments. Be aware of – and if you do not know, find out – who you can get to support your plans and possibly increase your resources. Resources means money, people (currently working elsewhere in a substance use service or at a basic, more infrastructural level), administration time and clinical space.

➤ Have an explicit but flexible plan that goes some way to accommodating some of the chaos resulting from substance use.

➤ Be mindful of succession planning within a skill mix while designing a service. For example, you may need to persuade commissioners that they should think in advance about the recruitment and retention of psychology staff during service design. Posts in remote and rural areas specialising in substance use are often difficult to fill. Career progression should be considered and built into a plan. Try to promote some of the transferability of skills from other areas such as adult mental health, public health and neuropsychological rehabilitation in job descriptions in order to widen the field of possible applicants for psychology posts. Be clear how you would use current skills and increase and develop knowledge in substance use.

➤ Consider how you could begin to use, and influence the use of, social cognitive theories to create behaviour change at a much wider societal level.[33,34]

➤ In the real world it is often a case of 'it's not what you're given, it's what you do with what you've got . . .'

CONCLUSION

This chapter began by asking readers to consider how to make best use of limited resources and to be reflective and creative in thinking about how to increase access to psychological interventions. It went on to describe the drivers and some of the challenges encountered in developing and increasing access to psychological services.

Simple or 'tame'[6] solutions can go some way to managing some of the technical or complicated challenges we come up against. However, the world in which we aim to design and deliver psychological services is complex and cuts across services and government departments. The micro and macro politics, values and relationships within organisations can hinder or block efforts to provide and increase access to services. Overnight, the resources and financial envelope available to fund psychological services can shrink to the size of a postage stamp, leaving what we have to work with much reduced. Uncertainty, losses, frequent changes and possible and actual conflict can affect professionals' personal resilience in attempting to progress services. There are many potential obstacles in the key learning points outlined in this chapter.

As professionals and service providers some of us will have natural talents and skills in managing the organisational challenges and opportunities that present when we are trying to develop services. Some of us will be less experienced and skilled.

We may need to draw on research, literature and thinking from outside our usual clinical sphere and comfort zones. The reading suggestions in this chapter can provide alternative ways of conceptualising and taking on challenges and opportunities. Gaining an understanding of complexity,[3–5,21–23] asking questions rather than presenting solutions to 'wicked' problems[6] and increasing our adaptive leadership skills[24–26] may go some way to supporting readers' efforts to increase access to psychological interventions.

REFERENCES

1 Si Kahn. 'It's not just what you're born with' song lyrics available at: http://sniff.numachi. com/pages/tiBORNWITH.html (accessed 18 October 2010).

2 King James Bible. Matthew 14:13-21.

3 Cooke-Davies T, Cicmil S, Crawford L, et al. We're not in Kansas anymore, Toto: mapping the strange landscape of complexity theory, and its relationship to project management. *Project Management Journal: Research Quarterly.* 2007; **38**: 50–61.

4 Murphy-Parker D, de Crespigny C. A perspective of nurse leadership and complexity theory; the international network of nurses (TINN) interested in alcohol, tobacco and drug misuse. *Drugs and Alcohol Today.* 2003; **3**(4): 5–11.

5 Obeng E. *New Rules for the New World: cautionary tales for the New World manager.* Mankato, MN: Capstone Publishing; 2001.

6 Grint K. Wicked problems and clumsy solutions: the role of leadership. *Clinical Leader.* 2008; **1**: 54–68.

7 National Institute for Health and Clinical Excellence. *Drug Misuse: psychosocial interventions. NICE Clinical Guideline 51.* London: NIHCE; 2007. http://guidance.nice.org.uk/ CG51. Also available at: www.nice.org.uk/nicemedia/live/11812/35975/35975.pdf (accessed 18 October 2010).

8 Scottish Intercollegiate Guidelines Network (SIGN). *The Management of Harmful Drinking and Alcohol Dependence in Primary Care: Guideline 74;* Edinburgh: SIGN; 2003. Available at: www.sign.ac.uk/pdf/sign74.pdf (accessed 27 September 2010).

9 Scottish Government. *The Road to Recovery: a new approach to tackling Scotland's drug problem.* 2008. Available at: www.scotland.gov.uk/Publications/2008/05/22161610/0 (accessed 27 September 2010).

10 Scottish Government. *Essential Care: a report on the approach required to maximise opportunity for recovery from problem substance misuse in Scotland.* Edinburgh: Scottish Advisory Committee on Drugs Misuse Integrated Care Project Group: Essential Care

Working Group; 2008. Available at: www.scotland.gov.uk/Resource/Doc/224939/0060866.pdf (accessed 27 September 2010).

11 Department of Health and National Treatment Agency for Substance Misuse. *The Effectiveness of Psychological Therapies on Drug Misusing Clients.* London: NTASM; 2005. Available at: www.nta.nhs.uk/uploads/nta_effectiveness_psycho_therapies_2005_rb11.pdf (accessed 18 October 2010).

12 Scottish Government. *Changing Scotland's Relationship with Alcohol: a framework for action.* Edinburgh; 2009. Available at: www.scotland.gov.uk/Publications/2009/03/04144703/0 (accessed 27 September 2010).

13 Department of Health and National Treatment Agency for Substance Misuse. *Drug Misuse and Dependence: UK guidelines on clinical management.* London: DOH; 2007. Available at: www.nta.nhs.uk/uploads/clinical_guidelines_2007.pdf (accessed 27 September 2010).

14 Department of Health, The National Institute for Mental Health in England, Care Services Improvement Partnership and The British Psychological Society. *New Ways of Working for Applied Psychologists in Health and Social Care: career pathways and roles.* London: DOH; 2007. Available at: www.bps.org.uk/the-society/organisation-and-governance/professional-practice-board/ppb-activities/new_ways_of_working_for_applied_psychologists.cfm (accessed 27 September 2010).

15 NHS Education for Scotland. *Delivering for Health and Applied Psychology: current workforce, future potential.* Edinburgh; 2006. Available at: www.scotland.gov.uk/Publications/2006/12/13130027/0 (accessed 6 February 2011).

16 NHS National Services Scotland. *Workforce Planning for Psychology Services in NHS Scotland: characteristics of the workforce supply in 2009.* Edinburgh: NHS Education Scotland and ISD publications; 2009. Available at: www.isdscotland.org/isd/6090.html (accessed 27 September 2010).

17 Royal College of Psychiatrists. *Availability of Psychological Therapies: a fair deal for mental health.* London: RCP; 2008. Available at: www.rcpsych.ac.uk/pdf/Fair%20Deal%20 manifesto%20(full%20-%201st%20July2009).pdf.pdf (accessed 27 September 2010).

18 Scottish Government . *Delivering for Mental Health: mental health and substance misuse: consultation draft.* Edinburgh; 2007. Available at: www.scotland.gov.uk/Publications/2007/06/29120532/0 (accessed 27 September 2010).

19 British Psychological Society. *New Ways of Working for Applied Psychologists in Health and Social Care: the end of the beginning.* Leicester: BPS; 2007. Available at: www.bps.org.uk/the-society/organisation-and-governance/professional-practice-board/ppb-activities/new_ways_of_working_for_applied_psychologists.cfm (accessed 18 October 2010).

20 Department of Health. *Commissioning Improving Access to Psychological Therapies for the Whole Community.* London: DOH; 2008. Available at: www.dh.gov.uk/en/Publications andstatistics/Publications/PublicationsPolicyAndGuidance/DH_090011 (accessed 27 September 2010).

21 Obeng E. *Putting Strategy to Work: the blueprint for transforming ideas into action.* London: Financial Times Pitman Publishing; 1996.

22 Obeng E. *All Change! The project leader's secret handbook.* London: Financial Times Pitman Publishing; 1996.

23 Obeng E, Gillet C. *The Complete Leader.* London: Pentacle Works the virtual media company in association with London Business Press; 2008.

24 Heifetz R. *Leadership Without Easy Answers.* Cambridge, MA: Belknap Press of Harvard University Press; 1994.

25 Heifetz R, Linsky M. *Leadership on the Line: staying alive through the dangers of leading.* Boston, MA: Harvard Business School Publishing; 2002.

26 Heifetz R, Grashow A, Linsky M. *The Practice of Adaptive Leadership: tools and tactics for changing your organization and the world.* Boston, MA: Harvard Business School Publishing; 2009.

27 British Psychological Society and Department Of Health. *Good Practice Guide on the Contribution of Applied Psychologists to Improving Access for Psychological Therapies*; 2007. Available at: www.bps.org.uk/the-society/organisation-and-governance/professional-practice-board/ppb-activities/improving_access_to_psychological_therapies.cfm (accessed 27 September 2010).

28 Mowbray D. *Review of Clinical Psychology Services.* Cheltenham: Management Advisory Service; 1989. Available at: www.mas.org.uk/uploads/articles/MAS%20Review%201989.pdf (accessed 18 October 2010).

29 Jones J, Weinberg L. Clinics for consultation and collaboration in learning disability services. *Clinical Psychology Forum.* 2006; **165**: 20–3.

30 Winstanley J. The Manchester Clinical Supervision Scale. *Nursing Standard.* 2000; **14**: 31–2.

31 McIntosh S. East Central Scotland Addictions Services Managed Care Network. *Psychological Services User Pathway (TIFF).* Tayside Psychological Services Unpublished. Available from the author.

32 Typpo M, Hastings JM. *An Elephant in the Living Room: a leader's guide for helping children of alcoholics.* Center City, MN: Hazelden Information and Education Services; 1984.

33 Patterson K, Grenny J, Maxfield D, *et al. Influencer: the power to change anything.* New York: McGraw-Hill; 2008.

34 Bandura A. Social cognitive theory goes global. *Psychologist.* 2009; **22**: 504–6.

TO LEARN MORE

- Learn more about leadership and project management: visit www.pentaclethevbs.com for links to Obeng's[5,21–23] work and www.vitalsmarts.com/influencer_book.aspx for resources and videos of master influencers at work (accessed 24 January 2011).
- Learn about social cognitive theory as a way of influencing behaviour change at a societal level. Useful references and links about Albert Bandura's[31] work available at: www.des.emory.edu/mfp/self-efficacy.html. Exciting work that has successfully used radio and television soaps and other media in different countries to influence behavioural change (sexual risk behaviours) at a societal level available at: www.populationmedia.org (accessed 24 January 2011).
- Buy the T shirt: 'I think you'll find it's a bit more complicated than that.' Available at: www.badscience.net – Goldacre B. *Bad Science.* London: Harper Collins; 2009 (accessed 24 January 2011).
- Goldsmith M. *What Got You Here Won't Get You There.* London: Profile Books; 2008. This book looks at habits (maybe even addictive behaviours) we have in relation to the behaviours and thinking we utilise in our approach to our work, and makes suggestions for change.
- McIntosh S. The development of East Central Scotland's Psychology Addictions Managed Care Network. *Poster Presentation at Conference: managed clinical networks, 10 years on.* Available from the author.
- National Treatment Agency for Substance Misuse. *Young People's Specialist Substance Misuse: exploring the evidence.* 2008. Available at: www.nta.nhs.uk/uploads/yp_exploring_the_evidence_0109.pdf (accessed 24 January 2011).
- Outhwaite S. The importance of leadership in the development of an integrated team. *Journal of Nursing Management.* 2003; **11**: 371–6.

- Scottish Executive Health Department. *Promoting the Development of Managed Clinical Networks in NHS Scotland.* Edinburgh: NHS HDL 69; 2002. Available at: www.sehd.scot.nhs. uk/mels/hdl2002_69.pdf (accessed 24 January 2011).
- Scottish Executive. *Mind the Gap: meeting the needs of people with co-occurring substance misuse and mental health problems.* Edinburgh; 2003. Available at: www.scotland.gov.uk/ Publications/2003/11/18567/29477 (accessed 24 January 2011).
- Scottish Executive. *A Fuller Life: report of the expert group on alcohol-related brain damage.* Edinburgh; 2004. Available at: www.scotland.gov.uk/Publications/2005/05/23141307/13104 (accessed 24 January 2011).
- Scottish Executive. *Building a Health Service Fit for the Future (The Kerr Report).* Edinburgh: NHS; 2004. Available at: www.scotland.gov.uk/Resource/Doc/924/0012112.pdf (accessed 24 January 2011).
- Scottish Executive. *Fair to All, Personal to Each: the next steps for NHS Scotland.* Edinburgh: NHS; 2004. Available at: www.scotland.gov.uk/Publications/2004/12/20400/48704 (accessed 24 January 2011).
- Scottish Government. *Getting the Right Workforce, Getting the Workforce Right.* Edinburgh: NHS; 2005. Available at: www.sehd.scot.nhs.uk/workforcedevelopment/publications/camh_ workforce_strategic_rev.pdf (accessed 24 January 2011).
- Scottish Government. *Delivery through Leadership: NHS Scotland leadership development framework.* Edinburgh: NHS; 2005. Available at: www.scotland.gov.uk/Publications/ 2005/06/28112744/27452 (accessed 24 January 2011).
- Scottish Government. *Hidden Harm – Next Steps: supporting children, working with parents.* Edinburgh; 2006. Available at: www.scotland.gov.uk/Publications/2006/05/05144237/0 (accessed 24 January 2011).
- Scottish Government. *The Matrix – Psychological Therapies: a guide to delivering evidence-based psychological therapies in Scotland.* 2008. Available at: www.bps.org.uk/dcp-scot/information- and-resources-for-professionals/delivering-psychological-therapies-the-matrix.cfm (accessed 24 January 2011).
- Scottish Government. *Towards a Mentally Flourishing Scotland: policy and action plan 2009–2011.* Edinburgh; 2009 Available at: www.scotland.gov.uk/Publications/2009/05/06154655/0 (accessed 24 January 2011).
- Sperlinger D, Davis P, Wanigaratne S. *Measuring Treatment Outcomes with Drug Misuse Clients.* Leicester: British Psychological Society and Centre for Outcomes Research and Effectiveness (CORE); 2003.

ACKNOWLEDGEMENTS AND THANKS
Acknowledgement and thanks to all the people who have helped with either improving access to psychological services across the managed care network or more directly in the writing of this chapter; in particular to Sam McGuire, Brian Kidd, Pam Gowans, Ian Taylor, Mike Hopley, Kirsty Gillings, Zoe Hughes, Marilyn Aitkenhead, Hazel Mackenzie, Alex Baldacchino, Lucy Cockayne, Peter Rice, Alison Hawitt, Iain, Cathie, Ben and Kiera McIntosh.

CHAPTER 4

Caring for the family

Alison Sadler

INTRODUCTION

Families can be destroyed by substance use. They are victims drawn into a world they cannot understand and do not want to be in. They find themselves dealing with abusive, deceitful and manipulative behaviour as the substance becomes all-important to the person. They cope with one nightmare situation after another as the person's life spirals out of control. Relationships are put under immense strain and the family suffers physically and mentally.

Mental health–substance use problems add another layer of complexity. With substance use alone there is always hope of recovery, but with mental health–substance use problems members of the family know that the chance of recovery is significantly reduced. Despite this, they show remarkable resilience and remain influential in the life of the individual experiencing the problems. Hope keeps them going, on a journey that can last many years.

SELF-ASSESSMENT EXERCISE 4.1

Time: 10 minutes
- Consider the concept of 'hope'.
- Is there a difference between 'hope' and 'expectation'?
- How can hope play a part in maintaining a strategy for the family's future?

SERVICES FOR FAMILIES

It has been difficult for families of individuals experiencing mental health–substance use problems to find appropriate support services. Even though they may provide considerable care to the individual, they often fail to recognise themselves as carers or make use of carers' services. Many have negative experiences of social services and will actively avoid them. Family members are usually employed and functioning adequately in society so they have no need of welfare services. Treatment services focus on the individual and have little to offer the family.

Consequently, their need for support has been hidden and only fulfilled when families have looked to one another and formed small support groups. The development of these groups across the country has been inconsistent, ranging from nothing available in some areas to dedicated, comprehensive services in others.[1]

ENGAGING WITH FAMILIES

Families do not engage easily; they feel stigmatised by society and want to keep their problems hidden (*see* Book 3, Chapter 2; Book 1, Chapters 4–7). To make contact with a support service takes a great deal of courage and if the first response is not right, the family will not engage and the opportunity is lost. It could be many years, if ever, before contact is made again.

Initial contact is most likely to be made when substance use is either suspected or discovered, or when the family reach a point of crisis. Often when families approach a support service their energy is totally focused on the individual and they can be reluctant to acknowledge that they themselves might benefit from support. It is only when they are asked about their own well-being that they can recognise the impact substance use is having on the whole family.

Supporting families can be based on the following five principles.

1 Provide information

When a family learns that not only does their relative have a mental health problem but also they are using substances, they are confused and frightened. They may have little knowledge of either condition and information can help them make some sense of their situation.

They might first turn to the professionals involved in the individual's care, but professionals can be reluctant to speak to the family, believing they risk compromising confidentiality. This is particularly true if the individual does not want the family involved. Families understand and respect the need for confidentiality, but general information about mental health–substance use problems can allay fears and answer some of their many questions. It also provides an opportunity to direct them to whatever local support services might be available.

Mental health and substance use services are not always well coordinated. Families can become frustrated as they find themselves passed from one speciality to another, trying to get information. This can be overcome if there is a liaison worker, knowledgeable in mental health–substance use problems and their complexities, available to talk with, and work alongside, the family.

There is sometimes an expectation that the family will be involved in the person's care simply because they live in the same house. Assumptions are made that they will take on such tasks as the supervision of medication, or participate in a home detoxification programme. Families rarely refuse; they will do whatever is required to help, but sadly these roles can be taken on with woefully little information or preparation. If the family's participation is required, the family members need to be fully informed and properly supported.

For some time, the family members may have been ignoring or rationalising strange behaviour because they have not understood its cause. Information about substances and recognising the signs of use can help them make distinctions between behaviour caused by substance use and that caused by mental illness. This knowledge gives the family more confidence to challenge unacceptable behaviour.

SELF-ASSESSMENT EXERCISE 4.2

> **Time: 10 minutes**
> * Consider what you might need to know/have, from a professional, if you were a family member.

Group learning can be beneficial for families as they have the opportunity to meet other families and share their experiences. Families are eager to learn anything that will strengthen their coping strategies, and inviting presentations from services and specialists gives them a greater understanding of the treatment system.

Information is empowering to families, enabling them to make informed choices; this reduces the feelings of helplessness and gives a sense of regaining control. It can dispel the many myths around mental health and substance use and help the family accept that their situation is not due to any action or omission on their part.

The need for information is ongoing as each new set of circumstances occurs, bringing with it new situations that can be totally out of the family's experience. They may need to ask previously unimaginable questions and they want frank and honest answers. Some statements made by the family can be found in Box 4.1.

BOX 4.1 Family statements

> 'Professionals always focused on mental health problems; no one seemed to address the substance misuse.'
> 'Doctors were only interested in his drinking; no one talked about the paranoia. One said there was nothing wrong.'
> 'We didn't realise there was help available for us. No one ever mentioned support for the family.'
> 'He could have saved me years of worry if he had given me more information.'
> 'We had very little knowledge of mental health issues or drugs; we learned through "Relatives of Drug Abusers".'

2 Give understanding and acceptance

Mental health–substance use problems affect every member of the family, and the individual consumes their lives. They become a safety net, stepping in when everything breaks down, to pick up the pieces once again. Their own lives are put on hold and their dreams and expectations are shattered.

Family members can be the ones who contact services on behalf of the individual, chase up professionals, make appointments and escort the individual to the door to make sure they get there. Family members take on a caring role, shopping, cleaning, washing and even monitoring personal hygiene. Even if the individual is living independently, the caring often continues. The family is likely to do whatever is necessary to try to prevent the individual from being evicted, this being a better option than taking her/him back into the family home. Some families try to budget for the individual in an effort to control the substance use and ensure bills are paid. Whatever they do to help financially, they may be pestered, persistently and constantly, for money.

One of the most difficult aspects for the family to deal with is erratic and unpredictable behaviour. The individual may be

➤ violent
➤ aggressive
➤ self-harming
➤ depressed
➤ suicidal

. . . and the family lives in dread of the next incident.

Society gives little recognition to the family's role. The professionals caring for the individual may not realise just what the family is coping with. In a psychiatrist's room, the individual may be reserved and compliant, very different from the belligerent, demanding, uncooperative person the family may battle with daily.

There is a tendency for society to blame problematic substance use on dysfunctional families, and there remains an underlying fear of mental illness. This can leave families feeling shamed and guilty, believing they are in some way to blame. Many react by becoming increasingly withdrawn and isolated; they have nowhere to go where they can feel understood and accepted without judgement.

Support groups provide a lifeline for many. Here families can rant and rave, laugh and cry, and voice thoughts and feelings they are unable to share anywhere else. They are supported and encouraged by others, close bonds are quickly made and additional support networks develop outside the group.

However, groups are not for everyone – for some, exposure in a group is too difficult to cope with. One-to-one, face-to-face meetings are an alternative and need not necessarily be with a professional; families welcome the opportunity to talk with others in similar situations. When families meet together they find the understanding and acceptance that eludes them elsewhere. Some statements on the difficulties faced by the family can be found in Box 4.2.

BOX 4.2 Family difficulties

'He came home so paranoid he would not go back for his possessions; I went for them and found the flat ripped apart.'

'The bank was giving him loans and credit; I had to battle to stop this happening but he can reapply at any time.'

'We are always dealing with the negative side of the behaviour; he will make an effort with other people, not with us.'

'It was 18 years before I went to a group. What an eye opener; I can laugh, chat, cry, swear and connect with others like me.'

3 Provide anonymity, discretion and confidentiality

Families can find themselves ostracised and even mistreated by their community. Long-term friends stop calling at the house, family members are shouted at in the street and the individual is accused of every theft and burglary in the neighbourhood.

To protect themselves, families can become incredibly adept at keeping their problems hidden. Friends, neighbours and work colleagues may not know what they are dealing with for many years. Extended family members are not told and in some cases even close family are unaware. A parent living away from the family home may not know that their child is experiencing substance use problems despite having regular contact. Concerns have simply been put down to adolescence, laziness or a bad attitude.

The fear of a negative reaction makes it difficult for a family to approach a support service, and when it does, many want to stay anonymous. Contact by telephone is the safest option and some families only ever engage in this way. They can choose not to give any personal details and if they feel threatened they can end the call and make no further contact.

Families may also want to avoid recognition when attending a support service. This can be difficult if the service is based at a treatment agency, as obvious conclusions can be drawn if they are seen. A shared-occupancy building reduces the risk of recognition and a home visit will avoid the issue, but discretion is still important if neighbours and other family members are unaware. Some may choose to meet in a public place or access a service outside their home area, although this can be a problem for the service if they have a contract that restricts the catchment area.

If family members are to feel safe they need a confidential service, and the service needs to be clear what this means. Confidentiality issues can be complex with family support if the individual is involved in illegal activities, and family members may have unwittingly committed offences by buying drugs or paying off dealers. They need to know that such information will not be passed to the authorities, but in the case of serious crime or child protection issues, this cannot be guaranteed. The service must have clear boundaries, with limits to its confidentiality policy that are clearly communicated to the family. Some statements expressing the feelings of desperation faced by the family can be found in Box 4.3.

BOX 4.3 Family desperation

'It was upsetting; I didn't want people to know.'

'Somehow mental was quite acceptable – he can't help it – but drugs was a shameful thing.'

'We are embarrassed; the neighbours have rejected us.'

'We feel helpless, desolate, isolated.'

4 Help families to refocus on their own lives

Families continue with their daily lives as best they can, but often at the expense of their own health and well-being. Tensions build among family members; relationships are torn apart and all too often there is separation and divorce. Stress, anxiety and depression are common, and related physical health problems can develop.

Families know that something has to change but all too often their efforts are focused on changing the individual. It can take a long time before family members realise they cannot force change; they can only influence it by changing their own behaviour. By refocusing on their own needs family members can reclaim a life of their own.

Some families will never come to this realisation, but others learn how to put emotional distance between themselves and the individual, stepping back to let the individual take responsibility for the choices she/he is making. If an individual chooses to spend rent money on drugs and is evicted, the family members learn to let them experience the consequences. Where once they might have rushed in to save the situation, they now hold back, which is difficult and painful to do. It is also complicated by mental illness as the individual's capacity to accept responsibility is reduced and their vulnerability makes it so much harder to witness the consequences.

Despite this, families affected by mental health–substance use problems do manage to put some basic rules in place and make the boundaries clear. For instance, a person may be invited to the family home every week if they agree to have a bath while there and refrain from smoking in the house. If they choose not to abide by these rules, the visits are stopped.

Many families give the individual money because it is easier to succumb to the constant demands than to cope with the conflict. This can cause considerable financial hardship, and once the family members start to refocus on their own needs they may make the decision to stop. Conflict is likely to escalate as the money is inevitably being spent on substances; ultimately, though, the family is setting a clear boundary that ends collusion and forces the person to take responsibility.

Families may also have to consider long-term financial implications. An inheritance can be potentially devastating for the individual, and families may need advice on setting up trust funds or specifying conditions of inheritance.

There will have been many disappointments over the years with holidays and special events ruined; relaxing and enjoyable family time may have disappeared completely. It may be no more than a walk, a coffee with a friend or attending a support group, but family members need to rediscover their own space. Regular respite and relaxation events can give this opportunity.

Putting some distance between themselves and the individual does not mean that family members no longer care. They may still choose to help and support but, when the focus shifts, they can find that there is life beyond substance use. Some statements made by family members relating to the impact of mental health–substance use can be found in Box 4.4

BOX 4.4 Family impact

'We asked him to leave after dealers started coming to the house demanding money; he got placed in a homeless hostel.'
  'I feel he has to know the rules.'
  'My only weapon is not to speak to him. He knows I'm upset then.'
  'We go away for weekends a lot; it's our escape.'
  'Hope keeps me going but it's a long road.'

5 Give families a voice

Families are experts in caring for the person experiencing substance use and mental health problems and, if they are listened to, they can make a valuable contribution to the treatment regime. Services do not always recognise the influence families have, because naturally they are focused on the individual. However, they could exploit this by working as equal partners. Professionals should not feel threatened by the family; both have the same priority – wanting the individual to access treatment and recover.

A collaborative agreement among the family, the individual and the professional can define terms of involvement and enable partnership working. When family members attend appointments, there is less opportunity for the individual to manipulate or deceive either party, and there are far fewer secrets – everyone is empowered.

The family may only require a small level of involvement but it can make an immense difference. When an individual is allowed to live at home only if they access treatment, the family needs to know they are attending appointments. If the individual is not attending, they are unlikely to tell the family. However, if the service confirms non-attendance, the family is empowered to enforce its boundaries.

Family involvement needs to be taken seriously. To invite family members to a case conference gives them a voice, but if they are never informed of the outcome or invited to attend again, it is meaningless. When a family is asked to work with the community team, members need to be regarded as part of that team and not ignored if changes are made to the service. Families find it difficult to challenge services because they fear it might jeopardise treatment, so family involvement needs to be offered routinely and the family treated as equal in the partnership.

SELF-ASSESSMENT EXERCISE 4.3

Time: 10 minutes
- Consider what you could do in practice to treat the family as equals.
- What might you need to change within your own practice?

Some services recognise how valuable families' views on treatment planning and service development can be and do encourage families to attend consultations. Unfortunately, representation is often low, not because families do not want to be heard but because they lack the time and energy to put themselves forward. To have an effective voice they need representatives with a genuine understanding of their needs who can speak on their behalf.

SELF-ASSESSMENT EXERCISE 4.4

Time: 10 minutes
- What other reasons can you think of as to why family members might not attend consultations?

- What could you do to facilitate/encourage attendance?
- What would you now need to do to your practice to implement such changes?

Drug treatment services are widespread throughout the UK but there are whole counties without a family support service. Those that are available tend to be small, underfunded charities or family support workers based in treatment agencies. The families' loudest voice is simply for adequate support services to be available for all families affected by substance use. Some statements supporting the benefits of family support are given in Box 4.5.

BOX 4.5 Family support

'Thank God for the support of his drugs worker. I am always welcome to join the meetings.'

'He says it as he sees it and then I tell it how it really is.'

'The worker sets goals for him, which is motivating. This support is an enormous help.'

'The social workers were helpful to my son but I wasn't included at all. I felt pushed out.'

MEETING THE ONGOING NEEDS OF THE FAMILY

Families are likely to access support over many years. They constantly fluctuate between times of crisis and calmer periods and this pattern influences how they use a support service. Some will access it regularly, finding ongoing support helps to keep them going; others will use the service every time there is a crisis and step back when the situation settles again.

The support offered needs to be flexible enough to respond to this. Families should have the option of attending groups regularly or intermittently, depending on their needs at that time. Telephone support may be required daily during a crisis but then contact may not be made again for months. If a family is looking for help, they do not want to be offered a support group meeting in two weeks' time or an appointment next week; they want and need an immediate response.

Support should also be tailored to the needs of different family members. A partner's focus may be on parenting and sexual health, whereas a grandparent caring for the individual's children may want information about legal and financial matters. Emotionally, men and women have different support needs, with men responding to a more factual approach while women may need more opportunity to express their feelings.

Families do not necessarily see themselves in need of care and/or want or need a treatment programme. Many would find it bewildering and perhaps even threatening to be offered a needs assessment or care plan at a first meeting. It has taken courage for them to risk contact and they want an informal, friendly and welcoming service.

This is not to say that structured interventions cannot be used with families. When trying to put boundaries in place with the individual, a family member might benefit from working towards a mutually defined action plan and goals. Families need to have the choice, and the introduction of a care plan needs to be timed appropriately.

When substance use stops, the family's need for support may continue. When a person is in recovery, the problems change rather than disappear. It is hard to trust that recovery will last as relapses are all too common, and the family has been hurt many times before. With mental health–substance use problems, the cessation of the substance use may intensify the mental health problems and increase the need for support.

Bereaved families can also continue to need support for a considerable time after the death. Bereavement through substance use has a painful and complicated grieving process. Family members struggle to come to terms with not only the death but also the wasted life and question what more they could have done to make a difference. Many find some comfort and understanding from other families bereaved through substance use.

SELF-ASSESSMENT EXERCISE 4.5

Time: 10 minutes
- What services exist in your geographical area that would offer support to the bereaved?
- How would you access such services?
- Make a list of useful contacts for future use.

CONCLUSION

The aim of this chapter has been to give an insight into the lives of families experiencing mental health–substance use problems and, by doing so, give an understanding of how best to support them.

The importance of caring for the family members cannot be overstated; they play a major role in the life and care of an individual experiencing mental health–substance use problems, and they are struggling daily for survival. If the family breaks down there are serious repercussions for everyone involved and for society.

Service commissioners are showing an increasing interest in family support as evidence is growing to show how influential the family is in encouraging the user to engage in treatment.[2]

This interest is welcomed but the development of any family support service must be primarily to support the family – any benefit for the individual is secondary. Families need and deserve services that are designed to meet their own needs.

REFERENCES

1 Adfam. *We Count Too: good practice guide and quality standards for work with family members affected by someone else's drug use.* 1st ed. London: Adfam; 2005. p. 15.
2 National Treatment Agency for Substance Misuse. *Supporting and Involving Carers: a guide for commissioners and providers.* 1st ed. London: National Treatment Agency for Substance Misuse; 2008. p. 7.

TO LEARN MORE

- Burton-Phillips E. *Mum, Can You Lend Me Twenty Quid? What drugs did to my family.* 1st ed. London: Piatkus; 2008.
- Cooper J, Cooper DB. Hope and coping strategies. In: Cooper J. *Stepping into Palliative Care: relationships and responses v. 1.* 2nd ed. Oxon: Radcliffe Publishing; 2006.
- Copello A, Velleman R, Templeton L. Family interventions in the treatment of alcohol and drug problems. *Drug and Alcohol Review.* 2005; **24**: 369–85.
- Dorn N, Ribbens J, South N. *Coping With a Nightmare: family feelings about long-term drug use.* 2nd ed. London: ISDD; 1994.
- Rubin C. *Don't Let Your Kids Kill You: a guide for parents of drug and alcohol addicted children.* Gardena, CA: SCB Distributors; 2007
- **Adfam** – www.adfam.org.uk – advice and practical guidance for groups and professionals working with families of substance misusers.
- **Frank** – www.talktofrank.com – information and advice on substances and services to individuals, their families, friends and carers.
- **PADA (Parents Against Drug Abuse)** – www.pada.org.uk – delivers support and services to the families of substance users across the country.
- **Rethink** – www.rethink.org – information and support for anyone affected by mental illness, including mental health–substance use problems.

ACKNOWLEDGEMENTS

I would like to acknowledge the contribution of families from RODA (Relatives of Drug Abusers) who are experiencing mental health–substance use problems and provided the quotes for this chapter.

CHAPTER 5

Caring for Indigenous people

Charlotte de Crespigny and Scekar Valadian

INTRODUCTION

This chapter describes the context of Indigenous Australians' poor general health, and particular factors influencing their alcohol, tobacco and other drug (ATOD) and mental health (MH) problems. It presents information about Indigenous peoples' holistic view of health and culturally respectful care. Screening, assessment and interventions for Indigenous people are discussed. Some key resources are provided regarding useful websites and additional reading.

TERMINOLOGY

The term 'Indigenous' encompasses all first-nation Australians, being the Aboriginal peoples of mainland Australia and Tiwi and Torres Strait islands.

HEALTH AND ILL HEALTH OF INDIGENOUS AUSTRALIANS

Health, according to the World Health Organization (WHO) is a state of complete physical, mental and social well-being, and a fundamental human right.[1] Indigenous Australians view health as the '*well-being of the whole community. This is a whole-of-life view and it also includes the cyclical concept of life-death-life*'.[2] As one of the oldest living cultures worldwide, Indigenous Australians have successfully survived in diverse environments over thousands of years. Since colonisation, adversity and life challenges have continued to impair their physical and mental health, yet their culture continues to survive and evolve.[3]

SELF-ASSESSMENT EXERCISE 5.1

Time: 10 minutes
- Consider your own culture, values and social norms.
- How might these differ from those of the Indigenous population?

Indigenous people are the poorest and sickest people in prosperous Australia. Life expectancy of non-Indigenous people is 17 years greater than that of Indigenous Australians.[4,5] The all-cause mortality rate of Indigenous Australians is twice that of

Māori, 2.3 times that of Native Americans and 3.1 times that of the total Australian population,[4,5] with many experiencing MH and ATOD problems.

The physical and mental ill health and ATOD problems of Indigenous people are directly linked to dispossession, racism and ongoing grief, poverty and cultural losses according to de Crespigny.[6,7] The Royal Australian and New Zealand College of Psychiatrists reported antecedents of mental distress as follows:

> Alienation, despair, depression, anxiety and psychosis all contribute to the use of substances in an attempt to escape or temporarily relieve symptoms. A social milieu of unemployment and mainstream hostility makes the abuse of substances in a community worse, and there is a powerful feedback loop through which the abuse of substances creates more misery for the abuser and for family and friends.[8]

Grief is frequently expressed through self-harm, suicide, ATOD dependence, mental illness, violence and abuse.[4,9] To recognise and respond effectively to such serious problems, health professionals must first acknowledge that cultural, spiritual and psychological trauma gravely affects Indigenous peoples' social, emotional, psychological and physical well-being.[7]

Cultural view of health

Indigenous cultures in Australia, while diverse in language and kinship groups, have mutual ways of understanding and experiencing life, death and well-being. A common belief is that health relies on having strong spiritual, cultural, psychological and physical well-being. The individual is inseparable from the family.[10]

Trauma and grief

Expressions of trauma and grief are various responses to deaths, distress, illness, ATOD dependence and self-harm. These are all too often experienced by family and friends in the context of incarceration and physical and mental abuse. Thus, the National Aboriginal Health Strategy Working Party stated: '*Mental distress is a common and crippling problem for many Aboriginal people and appropriate services are a pressing need.*'[10]

Swan and Raphael reiterated trauma and grief as

> among the most serious, distressing and disabling issues faced by Aboriginal people – both as a cause of mental health problems, and as major problems in their own right. They were seen as central to Aboriginal health and well-being. There is a need to provide educational, preventive, and clinical responses to address these ubiquitous issues.[8]

Childhood trauma is closely linked to transgenerational grief and poverty, particularly in the context of living in an affluent society. Therefore, Indigenous people need ready access to health promotion, harm reduction and early intervention programmes for their MH and ATOD problems. Swan and Raphael also strongly advised that

[s]ervices should be developed through specialised networks linked to child, adolescent and family therapy programmes in the general mental health services but ensuring that these are sensitive to and culturally informed about Aboriginal mental health.[8]

This advice has been taken up in some areas, but is yet to be systematically responded to.

KEY POINT 5.1

Family and kinship networks are fundamental to Indigenous life, making up the cultural and social environments in which Indigenous people live and raise their families. Sadly, many experience racism from service providers and professionals, resulting in alienation and reluctance to seek help or advice for their health or other concerns.

SELF-ASSESSMENT EXERCISE 5.2 (ANSWER ON P. 58)

Time: 5 minutes
- Consider what you could do to incorporate acceptable ways of acknowledging and welcoming Indigenous people.

ALCOHOL, TOBACCO AND OTHER DRUG (ATOD) USE

Worldwide, many people use alcohol, tobacco, pharmaceuticals and other psycho-active substances.[11] While ATOD use is common in the general population, it is less common among Indigenous Australians – other than tobacco.

We need to understand that people use ATODs for varying reasons as they serve a purpose.[12] Their experiences may or may not be problematic. People's ATOD experiences are influenced by individual characteristics, the physical and cultural environment[13] and the effects of the substance used.[12] For example, Saggers and Gray[13] describe the '*valued nature of drinking*' among various contemporary Indigenous community groups as '*seen by the drinkers themselves as an opportunity of socialising and enjoyment, and as a means of relieving boredom*'.[13]

Many Indigenous people who consume ATODs do so to relieve physical and emotional pain, hunger and bad memories.

Spectrum of ATOD problems

The spectrum of ATOD problems directly relates to the acute and longer-term effects of the drug, such as its depressant or stimulant effects on the central nervous system, and the pattern of consumption. Many Indigenous people who drink do so in groups, where purchasing and consumption can be shared, and drink for as long as funds last (e.g. several days). Some experience intoxication-related problems and others develop serious mental and physical illness, alcohol dependence and social problems.

SELF-ASSESSMENT EXERCISE 5.3 (ANSWERS ON P. 58)

> **Time: 10 minutes**
> - Consider and reflect on what you think are the types of ATOD problems people could experience.

Smoking cessation: a high priority

KEY POINT 5.2

Tobacco kills more Indigenous people than any other drug.

Given their extreme poor health, including high rates of cancer, lung and heart disease, diabetes and stroke, it is vital that every effort is made to assist Indigenous people to stop smoking. The Australian Bureau of Statistics (ABS) reported:

> In 2004–05, half the adult Indigenous population (50%) were current daily smokers . . . ABS health surveys record little change in the rate of smoking by Indigenous people since 1995 . . . For both men and women, smoking was more prevalent among Indigenous than non-Indigenous adults in every age group.[14]

Smoking cessation programmes need to be tailored, with healthcare providers working in collaboration with Indigenous services and interested community leaders. Indigenous smokers need ready access to education about the risks of smoking, proactive assistance, advice and resources for giving up, abstinence booster talks (phone and email) and free nicotine-replacement products.

Some smoking cessation programmes have already been adapted to suit Indigenous smokers, such as the *SmokeCheck*.[15]

SELF-ASSESSMENT EXERCISE 5.4 (ANSWER ON P. 58)

> **Time: 5 minutes**
> - Why is tobacco cessation such a high priority for Indigenous people?

CARING FOR INDIGENOUS PEOPLE

When caring for Indigenous people with ATOD and MH problems, Swan and Raphael advised:

> There is a need to encompass innovative frameworks, to provide for those with serious suffering and disability including all major mental disorders, and the interplay of these with comorbidity and consequences

of trauma and grief and substance abuse, for these are defined as critical and inextricably linked to mental health disorders.[8]

Mental health and ATOD health professionals in both general and specialist health services need to adopt the relevant cultural respect practices when working with Indigenous people.

Cultural respect in healthcare

Culturally respectful practice is critical to engaging, assisting and supporting Indigenous people. This does not require the professional to be an 'expert' on Indigenous culture. What is important is responding to cultural differences effectively and appreciating that these differences can affect one's perception and relationships with Indigenous people.[10]

SELF-ASSESSMENT EXERCISE 5.5

Time: 10 minutes
- Consider and reflect on how you can open yourself to learning more about the culture of Indigenous people.

Indigenous people have taught us the key elements of culturally respectful care. These involve **cultural awareness, cultural competence** and **cultural safety**.

Cultural awareness

This means understanding that cultural rules and values influence and sustain contemporary Indigenous societies. Health professionals must reflect on their own culture and values, and address any biases they have about Indigenous people.[10,16]

SELF-ASSESSMENT EXERCISE 5.6

Time: 10 minutes
- How might you acknowledge, and then address, any areas of cultural bias?

Cultural competence

This means offering effective care to an Indigenous person even though they have a different cultural background, and involves health professionals integrating their knowledge of Indigenous culture in interactions with the individual.[10,16]

Cultural safety

The Indigenous person needs to feel respected by the health professional and sense that they are safe. Any perceived cultural or power differences that exist need to be purposely diminished by the health professional.[10,17]

SELF-ASSESSMENT EXERCISE 5.7

Time: 15 minutes
- Think about the relationship (real or imagined) you make with an Indigenous person.
- Where does the balance of power lie?
- Does this balance of power differ from a community setting to an inpatient setting?
- Consider the difference and why this might be.

Spirituality and traditional healers

Indigenous people are strongly linked by spiritual connection to all things.[17] This provides them with the grounding, sense of purpose and space for healing so important in dealing with MH and ATOD problems.[10] Spirituality is the foundation of Indigenous peoples' identity and inseparably binds them to one another and their land (*see* Book 2, Chapter 13).

Many Indigenous people who seek healthcare also want access to their traditional ceremonies and bona fide (according to their community) traditional healers. This should be facilitated if at all possible.[9]

KEY POINT 5.3

Mental health is perceived as healthy spirit, and is central to Indigenous well-being. Understanding the importance of this connection for an Indigenous person experiencing ATOD and/or MH problems helps the healthcare professional to build rapport and trust. Respecting the individual's cultural connections and practices and offering them access to a traditional healer can be essential elements of healing.

SELF-ASSESSMENT EXERCISE 5.8 (ANSWER ON P. 59)

Time: 10 minutes
- Reflect on what you will need to help you learn about and deliver culturally respectful healthcare?

Comorbidities

Recent research indicates that over a five-year period of hospital admissions of Aboriginal people in South Australia individuals were diagnosed as having between 1 and 25 concurrent physical and MH–ATOD problems, the median being four. Diagnoses ranged across acute and chronic physical illnesses *in addition to* MH diagnoses. There was a strong association among ATODs, mental illness and preventable injury, with 25% having a concurrent head or other injury, poisoning or other consequences of external cause.[14] Likewise, many anecdotal stories from community members and health professionals emphasise the poor physical and mental health of many Indigenous people, and how seldom these complex health problems are treated holistically.

KEY POINT 5.4

Many Indigenous people who come to community clinics or hospitals have physical and mental health problems. They may also have ATOD problems directly or indirectly causing their ill health. It is essential to respond holistically so that multiple problems are considered. Clearly Indigenous people require integrated and well-coordinated approaches to screening, assessment, diagnosis and interventions.

ATOD PROBLEMS AND INTERVENTIONS
Alcohol screening

Next to tobacco, alcohol is the most serious drug problem among Indigenous people. However, unless specifically discussed, harmful drinking is frequently missed due to lack of systematic screening of all people aged 15 years and over. Many opportunities for early intervention and timely treatment are thus missed.

The Alcohol Use Disorders Identification Test (AUDIT) is used widely in Australia and elsewhere, having been developed and validated by the World Health Organization.[18,19] It can be administered as a brief written questionnaire for those sufficiently literate. It can also be administered via an interview, whereby the health professional asks the questions and scores the answers. Scores indicating likelihood of drinking problem and degree of risk (higher score = higher risk) require the health professional to then undertake a full assessment (*see* Table 5.1). AUDIT is not a diagnostic tool. Information on AUDIT and scoring is available at: http://whqlibdoc.who.int/hq/2001/who_msd_msb_01.6a.pdf (accessed 16 January 2011).

TABLE 5.1 AUDIT scores and assessment

Low risk	Risk	High risk
Score 0–7	Score 8–12	Score 13+
1–4 indicates low risk 5–7 indicates periods of intoxication	Indicates risk of short- and long-term harm to health	Indicates dependence
Provide advice on alcohol and its effects, and on harm reduction to prevent intoxication	10+ assess for tolerance/ risk of withdrawal Assess for other health and psychosocial problems Provide advice on alcohol and effects and harm reduction to prevent intoxication Include family as appropriate	Undertake comorbidity assessment, including physical and mental health Assess risk of withdrawal Assess for thiamine deficiency Assess for impaired cognition Assess for psychosocial problems Include family as appropriate

ATOD screening

While not specifically validated with Indigenous Australians, the Alcohol, Smoking and Substance Involvement Screening Test (ASSIST), can still be useful. Information on ASSIST is available at: www.who.int/substance_abuse/activities/assist/en/index.html (accessed 17 January 2011).

ATOD ASSESSMENT

Should screening indicate an ATOD problem the person needs to be fully assessed to determine the nature and seriousness of their use (*see* Chapters 8 and 9). This assessment should ideally be incorporated within the general health assessment and results documented therein.

An effective way of establishing the pattern of use is to work backwards from today for the last four weeks. Ask if this is the usual pattern and, if not, what usually happens. Table 5.2 can help to gather information about the pattern of ATODs used, amount/dose and route of administration, and reasons for use. A provisional diagnosis – for example, non-dependent or dependent – can then be attempted.

TABLE 5.2 ATOD assessment – ask from today's date

Drug	Amount	Frequency	Route	Who with	Periods of abstinence	Reason/s for use
Alcohol						
Tobacco						
Pituri (native tobacco)						
Prescribed medicines						
Over-the-counter medicines						
Traditional or herbal medicines						
Other drug/s						

Table 5.3 elicits information required for any acute presentation such as toxicity, overdose, withdrawal, injury or concurrent illness requiring medical treatment.

TABLE 5.3 Information required during acute presentation

Last use	Date:
	Time:
	Amount/dose:

Any changes in pattern over last 4 weeks

Blood alcohol level if intoxicated

Urine screen tests; other pathology results

Risk of imminent withdrawal

History of withdrawal seizures, hallucinations, delirium tremens, Wernicke's encephalopathy

History of accidental overdose/intentional overdose, toxicity, drug interactions; drug-induced psychosis; blood-borne viruses and other infections.

Figure 5.1 shows a flowchart of the responses needed according to problems revealed in assessment.

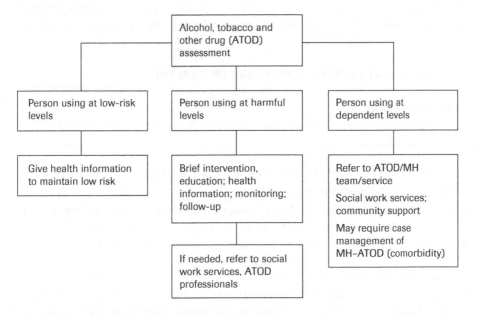

FIGURE 5.1 Responding to ATOD assessment findings[20]

RESPONDING TO PEOPLE WHO *ARE NOT* ATOD DEPENDENT

Many Indigenous people who **are not** dependent may experience problems of intoxication or more regular ATOD use but no serious comorbidities. Brief intervention for these individuals can be very effective (*see* Chapter 10; Book 4, Chapters 6–8).

SELF-ASSESSMENT EXERCISE 5.9 (ANSWERS ON P. 59)

> **Time: 10 minutes**
> The terms 'brief intervention' and 'early intervention' are often used interchangeably, even though there are differences in what we mean.
> • Note down what you think the differences might be.

Offering a brief intervention to the individual at a 'critical moment' while in hospital with a related injury or illness is often very effective in boosting willingness to reduce or stop ATOD use.[10,20,21]

KEY POINT 5.5

While those who are not dependent often respond well to brief intervention, those with dependence and more complex problems generally need more intensive and longer-lasting treatment. Information on early and brief interventions, motivational interviewing and harm reduction is available at: www.dassa.sa.gov.au/webdata/resources/files/ATOD_Clinical_Guidelines-book2.pdf – *see* Section 2.3, pp. 52–9 (accessed 17 January 2011).

SELF-ASSESSMENT EXERCISE 5.10 (ANSWERS ON P. 59)

> **Time: 5 minutes**
> • Which people do you think are *unlikely* to benefit from brief intervention?

TREATMENT OPTIONS FOR PEOPLE WHO ARE ATOD DEPENDENT
Using a person-centred approach

Interestingly, more Indigenous Australians give up dependent drinking than their non-Indigenous counterparts, and abstinence is often their preferred option. While harm reduction and controlled ATOD use may be available strategies, do not be surprised if abstinence is the individual's preferred goal.

Responding effectively to Indigenous people with dependence requires a personalised approach. Any treatment interventions should be carefully selected based on the ATOD diagnosis, and be explained in a language understood by the individual or by an interpreter. The treatment plan should be made in full consultation with the individual and, if possible, their chosen family members.

It is essential that the individual's capacity (cognitive and psychosocial) is assessed and determined. This will avoid involving people in programmes that they are unable to manage or benefit from,[10] such as having alcohol-related brain injury. These individuals are likely to need support for daily living and specialised programmes that offer structure and activities that support abstinence. They also require regular monitoring of their physical and mental health.

SELF-ASSESSMENT EXERCISE 5.11

Time: 10 minutes
- Consider therapies that might be helpful in maintaining physical and mental well-being.

If able and willing, there are useful therapies that the dependent individual, even with MH problems, can benefit from. Therapies may be offered in combination and include:
➤ pharmacotherapy (*see* Chapter 13)
➤ grief and other counselling
➤ anger management
➤ narrative therapy
➤ cognitive behavioural therapy (*see* Chapters 11 and 12; Book 4, Chapter 10)
➤ inpatient and outpatient rehabilitation.

KEY POINT 5.6

Reading or listening to stories of other Indigenous people who have overcome their ATOD dependence appears to be helpful both as a motivator for change and as encouragement 'along the way'. This book may help the individual: Brady M. *Giving Away the Grog: Aboriginal accounts of drinking and not drinking.* Canberra: Australian Government Department of Health and Ageing; 2005. Available at: www.alcohol.gov. au (accessed 17 January 2011).

With inpatient treatment, Indigenous people generally prefer to be near their family and country. If this is not possible, they may manage if they have regular contact with family members. This can be through regular visits, mail, phone, email, computerised phone calls and so forth.

Choice of treatment
There are no clear rules about whether Indigenous people who are substance dependent should be treated by primary healthcare or specialist services, either locally or away from home. Treatment modality should be based on the severity of dependence, their mental and physical health and personal preferences. These may include:
➤ grief counselling, ATOD therapy and supportive care
➤ treatment with a general practitioner in consultation with specialist services
➤ shared care among local Indigenous health service, community MH and drug and alcohol teams
➤ pharmacotherapy, counselling and/or rehabilitation in specialist ATOD or MH services.

KEY POINT 5.7

Many individuals and family members believe that detoxification is a treatment and wonder why there has not been a 'cure'. It is important that the individual understands that detoxification **is not a treatment in itself** but is rather the process of physically clearing ATODs from the body in preparation for treatment and rehabilitation, or as a short-term break from use.

Pharmacotherapy

Indigenous people may be unaware of pharmacotherapy and need to be informed about how they may benefit. Depending on the drug used, the individual may be eligible for:
➤ methadone or buprenorphine for opioid dependence
➤ nicotine-replacement therapy for nicotine dependence
➤ acamprosate or naltrexone for alcohol dependence.

These medications may or may not be prescribed in combination with other medications for their MH or other condition.[10] Health professionals and community members have reported anecdotally that these treatments are beneficial for many Indigenous people.

Coming home

Returning-to-home programmes and local support services are necessary for Indigenous people who have undertaken rehabilitation away from their community. Health professionals, individuals and families need to discuss and plan for this from the start of treatment. Skills development and practical strategies are needed to enable the person to adapt to a new life at home without ATODs. This will need family and health professionals to help with relapse prevention and management (*see* Book 4, Chapters 4 and 13; Book 6, Chapters 15 and 16), and other challenges that will arise.

SCREENING FOR ATOD AND MH COMORBIDITY

Due to the high prevalence of complex health issues faced by Indigenous people, many are at risk of ATOD and MH problems. The Indigenous Risk Impact Screen (IRIS) tool is unique in that it was developed and validated **specifically** for Indigenous Australians. It screens for alcohol, tobacco, other drug *and* mental health problems. For access to **IRIS, its scoring processes** and other information see: *Alcohol Treatment Guidelines for Indigenous Australians, Chapter 4: Alcohol and mental health problems.* Australian Department of Health and Ageing. 2007. pp. 11.130–11.145. Available at: www.alcohol.gov.au/internet/alcohol/publishing. nsf/Content/AGI02 (accessed 17 January 2011). This material is copyright free.

Assessing ATOD and mental health

If the IRIS score is indicative of ATOD and MH problems, it is necessary to undertake a full clinical assessment to determine what treatment options and care plan might be appropriate.

KEY POINT 5.8

Health professionals with minimal specialist training should exercise caution if undertaking ATOD and MH assessment and treatment. Liaison and close consultation with specialist services is strongly advised.

Shared care and managing ATOD and MH

ATOD and MH problems need to be treated concurrently rather than sequentially. Taking a longer-term perspective is also needed as complex problems are not likely to resolve quickly or easily. A 'shared care' approach involving the primary health professionals and specialist ATOD and MH professionals is advised.

Shared care can be undertaken directly or by remote means, depending on where the person lives, their capacity to manage, their family's capacity, and availability and accessibility of services. By using an integrated approach to assessment, care planning, treatment and follow-up care, many people can stabilise and improve.

A long-term perspective and taking a realistic, person-centred approach is useful for both parties.

Empowerment

Asking about MH is as important as asking the Indigenous person about his/her physical health. Educate, identify and manage problems together:
➤ identify what they perceive as their main concerns
➤ educate and support them in managing medications safely
➤ set realistic goals
➤ build confidence that they can achieve their goals
➤ take small, achievable steps
➤ have hope that there are ways to change behaviours
➤ learn that lapses may occur
➤ learn skills of relapse prevention and management
➤ access services and resources – for example, housing, education, employment, financial guidance, self-help groups.

Relapse

When people experience ATOD and MH problems, even when managing well, there can be occasions when there is worsening of symptoms. Such re-emergence of symptoms may be due to the nature of the condition and/or resumption of ATOD use. These issues need to be considered when planning treatment and aftercare, with the individual being supported and closely monitored.

KEY POINT 5.9

Families need to be fully informed about how to recognise early warning signs and when to seek help. It is imperative that comprehension is assessed frequently and clarifications made as required.

Working with the family

It is important health professionals recognise that in any community Indigenous people will maintain strong cultural ties with family. Traditional kinship rules may determine who can give and receive information about a family member, and who can make decisions on behalf of another (*see* Chapter 4; Book 3, Chapter 2; Book 4, Chapter 2). An Indigenous person may present to the service alone or with one or more family members, and this needs to be welcomed.[10] Building a respectful relationship with the individual and family, and maintaining flexibility, enables the health professional to help individuals overcome fear or other barriers to accessing information, treatment and support, by:

➤ enabling family or others to stay with the individual if requested
➤ supporting a preferred family member to attend during the assessment, and related discussions.[10]

Education should also be offered to family members where possible. It is important that the information is culturally acceptable. It should include drugs and effects, risks, various health conditions that can occur and the range of strategies and services that can help. Offer time for individual and family members to ask questions and discuss their options for better health. There is a wide range of pictorial and printed information available to assist people in making decisions about their ATOD use.

These websites may be of interest:
➤ www.adac.org.au (accessed 17 January 2011).
➤ www.adca.org.au (accessed 17 January 2011).
➤ www.alcohol.gov.au/internet/alcohol/publishing.nsf/Content/resources-menu ?OpenDocument&CATEGORY=Aboriginal+and+Torres+Strait+Islander+He alth+products&SUBMIT=Search (accessed 17 January 2011).

Effective referral

When referral is required, the health professional should offer information about the new service and what to expect. The individual may also require help in getting to appointments. Enhance uptake of referral by putting the person in direct contact with the new service provider/professional by telephone while she/he is with you. This can build confidence and willingness to proceed.[10]

Follow-up

Regular health check-ups and feedback improves effectiveness of treatment. Offering regular follow-up even when the individual has been referred on indicates that the professional cares about his/her well-being. It also provides the individual with the opportunity to obtain further support if needed, and assists with relapse prevention and management.

Reducing harm

The skills and resources to reduce risks and harm must be offered to all people with ATOD and MH problems, whether or not they are able or ready to stop or reduce use. The health professional will provide advice on anticipating and reducing risks from a range of situations; for example:

➤ intoxication
➤ drink driving
➤ sharing injecting equipment
➤ mixing alcohol or drugs with prescribed or other medications.

Knowing about local issues

It is useful to consult Indigenous services and community leaders to obtain information about local ATOD and MH issues. Accessing local reports and media accounts provides a 'picture' of the issues influencing the Indigenous community, and reveals what Indigenous people and their families could be personally experiencing.

RISK OF SUICIDE OR SELF-HARM

People who are intoxicated, depressed or experiencing other serious MH problems are at significant risk of suicide or self-harm. The immediate risk needs to be assessed so that urgent identification and attention occurs. This risk assessment must be part of the general assessment, no matter how well the person is known or what the health professional believes to be their current situation.

KEY POINT 5.10

If an individual is at risk, **seek expert advice immediately. Be prepared** – have an up-to-date emergency contact list nearby **in advance**.

The individual, and the family, must be informed that immediate help and specialist advice are being sought on their behalf, and that urgent transfer and admission to an acute-care hospital is highly likely. **For a useful suicide prevention resource** refer to Suicide Questions, Answers and Resources (SQUARE), a suicide prevention resource for health professionals, available from the Living Is For Everyone (LIFE) website at: http://livingisforeveryone.com.au (accessed 17 January 2011).

CONCLUSION

Being comfortable in your professional role is important when working with Indigenous people. Health professionals need not be constrained in offering information and intervention to Indigenous people with MH and ATOD problems. Being culturally respectful towards the individual and family builds trust and willingness to seek help for immediate and longer-term care.

POST-READING EXERCISE 5.1 (ANSWERS ON PP. 59–61)

Time: 30 minutes

Case study

Harry is an older Indigenous man living in a rural community with his family. His sister has brought him to your service, as she is worried about his health and spirit. He is not sleeping well and seems sad and ill. He has diabetes. He has been drinking wine every day since his wife died a year ago. Before that, Harry was abstinent for many years. Harry seems uncomfortable when you talk to him because he does not look at your face and only nods his head when you ask him questions. His sister tells you she wants to stay with him and seems comfortable talking to you.

1 List the outstanding problems Harry is faced with.
2 How will you approach Harry?
3 What do you need to do to?
4 How will you involve his sister?
5 How will you approach his screening and assessment?
6 What might his ATOD problem/s be?
7 Who else might you consult?
8 What do you need to consider when developing his care plan?

REFERENCES

1 World Health Organization. *Report of the Proceedings of the Conference Held at Alma Ata.* Ontario, Canada: WHO; 1978.

2 National Aboriginal Health Strategy. *Ways Forward: National Aboriginal and Torres Strait Islander Mental Health Policy National Consultancy Report; a national Aboriginal health strategy* (1989). Canberra: Commonwealth of Australia; 1989. p. 2.

3 Australian Health Ministers' Advisory Council. *Cultural Respect Framework for Aboriginal and Torres Strait Islander Health, 2004–2009.* Australian Health Ministers' Advisory Council. Standing Committee on Aboriginal and Torres Strait Islander Health Working Party. Commonwealth of Australia. Published by Department of Health South Australia. March; 2004. p. 4.

4 Gallaher G, Ziersch A, Baum F, *et al. In Our Own Backyard: urban health inequities and Aboriginal experiences of neighbourhood life, social capital and racism.* Adelaide: Flinders University; 2009.

5 Council for Aboriginal Reconciliation. *The People's Movement for Reconciliation: proceedings of the Australian Reconciliation Convention.* Kingston, ACT; 1997. Available at: http://trove. nla.gov.au/work/7395557?selectedversion=NBD22687838 (accessed 28 September 2010).

6 de Crespigny C. Double jeopardy: disadvantage and drug problems. *Australian Journal of Primary Health.* 2002; **8**: 70–6.

7 Royal Australian and New Zealand College of Psychiatrists. Submission to the House of Representatives Standing Committee on Family and Community Affairs. In: *Double Jeopardy: disadvantage and drug problems.* Canberra: Commonwealth of Australia; 2000.

8 Swan P, Raphael B. *Ways Forward: National Aboriginal and Torres Strait Islander mental health policy National Consultancy Report.* Canberra: Commonwealth of Australia; 1995. p. 9.

9 Australian Government Department of Health and Ageing. *Alcohol Treatment Guidelines for Indigenous Australians*. Canberra: Commonwealth of Australia; 2007. p. 10. Available at: www.health.gov.au/internet/alcohol/publishing.nsf/Content/AGI02 (accessed 28 September 2010).

10 *National Aboriginal Health Strategy 1989*. Canberra: Commonwealth Department of Health and Ageing; 1989. p. 171. Available at: www.quitnow.info.au/internet/main/publishing.nsf/Content/health-oatsih-pubs-NAHS1998 (accessed 18 October 2010).

11 Zinberg N. Drug, *Set and Setting: the basis of controlled intoxicant use*. New Haven: Yale University Press; 1984.

12 Brady M. *Giving Away the Grog: Aboriginal accounts of drinking and not drinking*. Canberra: Australian Government Department of Health and Ageing; 1995.

13 Saggers S, Gray D. *Dealing with Alcohol: Indigenous usage in Australia, New Zealand and Canada*. Cambridge: Cambridge University Press; 1998. p. 79.

14 Australian Bureau of Statistics (ABS). *National Aboriginal and Torres Strait Islander Health Survey, 2004–05*. Canberra: ABS; 2006. Available at: www.abs.gov.au/AUSSTATS/abs@.nsf/Lookup/4715.0Main+Features12004–05?OpenDocument (accessed 28 September 2010).

15 SmokeCheck. *Smoking Cessation Guidelines for Australian General Practice: practice handbook*. 2004 ed. Available at: www.quitsa.org.au/cms_resources/documents/Australian GeneralPracticeGuidelineHandbook.pdf (accessed 28 September 2010).

16 MacKean J. Personal comment. Adelaide, South Australia; 2005.

17 Kowanko I, de Crespigny C, Murray H. *Better Medication Management for Aboriginal People with Mental Health Disorders and Their Carers: final report*. Adelaide: Flinders University; 2003.

18 Babor T, Higgins-Biddle J, Saunders J, *et al. The Alcohol Use Disorders Identification Test: guidelines for use in primary care*. 2nd ed. Geneva: World Health Organization; 2001.

19 Saunders J, Hall W, Conigrave K. *Development of the Alcohol Use Disorders Screen Test (AUDIT): WHO collaborative project on early detection of persons with harmful alcohol consumption II*. Addiction. 1993; 88: 791–804.

20 de Crespigny C, Talmet J, Modystack K, *et al. Alcohol, Tobacco & Other Drugs: guidelines for nurses and midwives; clinical guidelines*. Version 2. Adelaide: Flinders University and Drug and Alcohol Services Council South Australia; 2003.

21 Heather N, Rollnick S, Bell A, *et al.* Effects of brief counselling among male heavy drinkers identified on general hospital wards. *Drug and Alcohol Review*. 1996; **15**: 29–38.

22 Lovibond SH, Lovibond PF. *Manual for the Depression Anxiety Stress Scales*. 2nd ed. Sydney: Psychology Foundation; 1995.

TO LEARN MORE

- Brady M. *The Grog Book: strengthening indigenous community action on alcohol*. Canberra: Australian Government Department of Health and Ageing; 2008.
- Brady M. Historical and cultural roots of tobacco use among Aboriginal and Torres Strait Islander people. *Australian and New Zealand Journal of Public Health*. 2002; **26**: 120–4.
- Brady M. *First Taste: how Indigenous Australians learned about grog. Set of six resources*. Canberra: Alcohol Education and Rehabilitation Foundation and Australian National University, Goanna Print Canberra; 2008.
- de Crespigny C, Kowanko I, Murray H, *et al.* A nursing partnership for better outcomes in Aboriginal mental health, including substance use. *Contemporary Nurse*. 2006; **22**: 275–87.
- Kowanko I, de Crespigny C, Murray H, *et al.* Better medication management for Aboriginal people. *Aboriginal & Islander Health Worker Journal*. 2004; **28**: 11–13.

- Kowanko I, de Crespigny C, Murray H, *et al*. Improving Indigenous health through better medication management: an overview. *Australian Journal of Primary Health*. 2005; **11**: 17–23.
- Office for Aboriginal and Torres Strait Islander Health Australian Government Department of Health and Ageing. *Evaluation of the Bringing Them Home and Indigenous Mental Health Programs: final report*. Canberra: Commonwealth of Australia; 2007.
- *Health is Life: report on the inquiry into Indigenous health*. Canberra: House of Representatives Standing Committee on Family and Community Affairs; 2000. Available at: www.aph.gov.au/House/committee/fca/indhea/reportfinal.pdf (accessed 28 September 2010).
- Australian Indigenous HealthInfoNet Available at: www.healthinfonet.ecu.edu.au/ (accessed 23 January 2011).
- National Indigenous Drug and Alcohol Committee (NIDAC) Available at: www.nidac.org.au/ (accessed 23 January 2011).
- *Alcohol Treatment Guidelines for Indigenous Australians*. Available at: www.health.gov.au/internet/alcohol/publishing.nsf/Content/AGI02 (accessed 23 January 2011).
- Indigenous risk impact screen (IRIS) and brief intervention (alcohol, tobacco, other drugs and mental health problems) Available at: www.health.qld.gov.au/atod/prevention/iris.asp#irismaterials (accessed 23 January 2011).
- Drug and Alcohol Services SA. Available at: www.dassa.sa.gov.au (accessed 23 January 2011).
- National 'Beyondblue' mental health resource. Available at: www.beyondblue.org.au (accessed 23 January 2011).

ANSWER TO SELF-ASSESSMENT EXERCISE 5.2

By doing this Indigenous people will come to know and trust you and be willing to seek your assistance. They will feel that being Indigenous is respected and that you genuinely wish to be of service.

ANSWERS TO SELF-ASSESSMENT EXERCISE 5.3

- One-off or occasional intoxication
- Regular harmful use
- Dependence
- People may experience work, relationship and social problems
- The ATOD use may be exacerbated or cause serious physical and MH problems or premature death

ANSWER TO SELF-ASSESSMENT EXERCISE 5.4

Smoking causes more premature death and chronic illness among Indigenous people than any other drug.

ANSWER TO SELF-ASSESSMENT EXERCISE 5.8

To deliver culturally respectful care, healthcare professionals need specific time, education and support. This is important for drug, alcohol and MH professionals.

ANSWERS TO SELF-ASSESSMENT EXERCISE 5.9

- *Early intervention* aims to intervene as early as possible in the person's ATOD and/or MH problem, however serious, in order to interrupt the trajectory of problems.
- *Brief intervention* is a 'one-off' or several brief counselling sessions offering information, advice and strategies to assist a person to address their non-dependent ATOD issues.[22]

ANSWERS TO SELF-ASSESSMENT EXERCISE 5.10

- ATOD dependence
- Serious physical illness and ATOD
- Possible MH problems and ATOD

ANSWERS TO POST-READING EXERCISE 5.1

1 Harry is elderly with multiple physical, social and emotional issues. He is living in a rural area, which has meant that, apart from his sister, who also has significant health problems, he has limited overall health and social support. He is grieving for his wife and drinking alcohol as a way of trying to dull his emotional pain. The grief and effects of alcohol may both be contributing to his poor sleep, depression and 'lost spirit'. Clearly, before his wife died Harry had not been drinking. His demeanour may reflect shame about his situation and/or be symptoms of his depression. It may be because he does not know you or what to expect from this encounter. Clearly, his diabetes and general health, as well as his mental health and drinking, need to be attended to holistically. His sister will be a great help in working with you and Harry, providing this is what he wants. Invite her to stay with him and contribute to his assessment and care.

2 It is important to make sure Harry is informed of your name and role, the nature of your service and that you are there to help. As he is not looking directly at you (no direct eye contact), place yourself slightly to one side so you both look forward rather than at each other while you converse. Ask Harry if he requires any help today such as housing or other social support as this may be preventing him from relaxing and focusing on his 'sadness' depression and drinking right now. If there are issues that require more immediate attention offer to liaise and establish how his needs can be met before proceeding with your assessment and care planning.

3   You need to build rapport and trust with Harry and his sister. They need to feel respected and confident that you are there to help and that you will consider their particular situation. Due to his presentation, you first need to assess Harry's immediate needs today. These will require attention before you can progress to any in-depth assessment and adequate identification (diagnosis) of his alcohol and MH status. Make sure he is comfortable, not intoxicated or at risk of withdrawal and therefore requiring medical/nursing supervision, that any prescribed medications are being managed appropriately, particularly his diabetes regime, and that he is stable socially. You may be able to move into full assessment during this initial visit, or alternatively arrange for him to return as soon as practicable once his more immediate needs have been attended to.

4   Introduce yourself to Harry's sister. The fact that she has come with him suggests this is his preference and that she is likely to play a prominent role in this encounter and his overall care. Let them both know that she is welcome and invite her to assist when and as she feels it is appropriate. Let them both know that the conversation is private but that you may need to share some health information with the treating team such as the diabetes and MH professionals.

5   Be aware that an Indigenous person like Harry may have different cultural understandings and ways of expressing sadness (depression) or anxiety – that is, 'lost his spirit' as well as the meaning of his alcohol use.[9] These issues will need to be raised and discussed and clarified with Harry and/or his sister so that you can make a more informed assessment of his presentation and treatment needs.

Undertake the interview version of the AUDIT questionnaire to determine Harry's drinking pattern and likely risk level, followed by a comprehensive alcohol and other drug assessment. While there is no validated depression scale that we have identified for Indigenous people in Australia there may be one elsewhere. Otherwise use the Lovibond and Lovibond (1995) DASS Scale (abbreviated 21-item version),[23] which measures active depression, anxiety and stress scales concurrently. This is available in the public domain.

Depending on his screening-results score and results from his in-depth assessment, you will need to talk to Harry and his sister about available treatment and support that they may consider. Inform Harry of his options, and how you can support holistic care that includes his diabetes, medication management and any other health problems.

6   Alcohol dependence; depression due to grief and possibly a pharmacological affect of excessive alcohol; sleep problems, which may be due to unsafe or noisy living conditions and/or his alcohol consumption and depression. Diabetes and possibly other health problems that may or may not have been diagnosed and need to be reviewed and an updated treatment plan.

7   You will need to consult the key worker of his local Indigenous health service or his general practitioner and other health professionals involved in treating his diabetes and any other health problems. You will also need to liaise with other services that may be assisting him with his general living and social needs. Once you have consulted these groups you will be able to formulate his care plan from your perspective.

8   It will be essential to work with Harry's sister and any other people involved in

his care so as to maximise his well-being, help him manage his physical and MH issues and stop drinking. It is also important to consider Harry's mental and physical capacity to undertake complex changes in his day-to-day life. He is sick, sad and elderly, and may have some cognitive dysfunction that will limit his capacity to benefit from, for example, cognitive behavioural therapy – and this will need to be considered.

He may benefit from regular structured activities and support such as attending alcoholics anonymous (AA) meetings. Cultural support including his choice of music may assist him to relax and sleep better, and feel more positive. Joining a local Aboriginal men's or mixed group may be helpful if and when he feels more able to socialise.

A medically prescribed and supervised acamprosate regime may assist him in maintaining alcohol abstinence, and depending on his MH diagnosis, other prescribed medications such as an antidepressant may be useful at least in the short term. Depending on his consumption pattern and tolerance to alcohol, he may require planned detoxification in hospital where his withdrawal and diabetes can be managed effectively. He will require 100 mg oral thiamine daily for prevention of Wernicke's encephalopathy, and additional nutritional support to maximise his diabetes management and overall health.

It is likely that Harry may require longer-term health monitoring and social support, and this needs to be considered within his holistic treatment and referral plan.

CHAPTER 6

Early intervention with young people

Ian Wilson

INTRODUCTION

There is a growing awareness of the needs of people who have problems with their mental health and who are also using substances. Traditional service approaches have been questionable, with problems of engagement and a lack of consistent and accurate detection and assessment. Many of the attitudes and values displayed by professionals have been unhelpful in engaging individuals in treatment, with some services having restrictive gate-keeping criteria leading to exclusion and marginalisation of some of the most vulnerable individuals. However, there are now some good examples of effective practice in joint working and the development of high-quality integrated and specialist services.

KEY POINT 6.1

In the UK, issues around mental health–substance use are among the most important for modern mental health services to address.

Professionals now regularly attempt to engage this challenging group in addressing not only their mental health needs but also their substance use.

This chapter will summarise the developing evidence base for effective working alongside people experiencing mental health–substance use problems. It will explore issues of mental health–substance use when working alongside people experiencing a first or recent onset of psychosis, by looking at ways of influencing professional attitudes and values towards these individuals and helping to enhance knowledge and skills. Practical ways will be suggested for engaging young people with a first or recent onset of mental distress who are using substances. A case study is offered to illustrate some of the principles of applying evidence-based practice.

PREVALENCE RATES IN ADULT MENTAL HEALTH AND SUBSTANCE USE SERVICES

Prevalence rates of mental health and substance use problems are high, in both mental health and substance use services. Substance use in the psychiatric population is in excess of 50%. Lifetime prevalence of mental health–substance use is as high as 47% in those individuals with a diagnosis of schizophrenia, 84% in those with personality disorders and 32% in those experiencing an affective disorder.[1] Rates of substance use appear to be higher among people experiencing severe mental illness (SMI) than in the general population.[2] In the UK, the prevalence of mental health–substance use ranges from 20% to 70%.[3] Around 16% of people using mental health services use alcohol to excess.[4] The prevalence estimate for current cannabis use in mental health services is 23%.[5] Lifetime use rate is 42.1%. Working alongside people experiencing mental health–substance use problems has, therefore, become a routine part of mental healthcare.[6] People undergoing substance use treatment also have high rates of mental ill health. Twenty-six per cent of drug treatment users and 46.8% of alcohol treatment users suffer from severe depression. The figures are 19% and 32.3% for severe anxiety, while 7.9% of drug treatment users and 19.4% of alcohol treatment users have a psychosis.[7]

MENTAL HEALTH–SUBSTANCE USE AND EARLY INTERVENTION

High rates of substance use are reported in individuals entering mental health services for the first time. For instance, 37% with first-episode psychosis met the criteria for drug use, drug misuse and alcohol misuse.[8] Substance use in people with first-episode psychosis has been reported as being twice that of the general population.[9] Those most at risk of substance use in this group were young males.

PATTERNS OF DRUG USE IN THE UK

The use of substances is a worldwide issue.[10] However, the UK appears to have a bigger problem than many other countries – the numbers of people using drugs are among the highest in Europe. According to the British Crime Survey 2008/9,[11] more than a third (36.8%) of 16- to 59-year-olds have used one or more illicit drugs in their lifetime, around one in ten (10.1%) in the last year.[11]

KEY POINT 6.2

Cannabis is the most widely used illicit substance in Europe[12] and the UK.

There are approximately 3.5 million users of cannabis, with cocaine, ecstasy and amphetamines being the next most popular illicit drugs.

WHY DO YOUNG PEOPLE TAKE DRUGS?

SELF-ASSESSMENT EXERCISE 6.1

Time: 10 minutes
- Think of some of the reasons why young people take drugs.
- Make a list – see how many you come up with.

The reasons why young people choose to use drugs are many and varied.[13] They can be seen as enjoyable, and they are freely available and relatively cheap (the price of various drugs appears to have been falling steadily and this is also true of alcohol). People also take substances because they are curious about the effects and because they are bored with their lives. Some young people use substances because they can change how they feel, often in a more 'predictable' manner than other things in their lives. For instance, if a young person is feeling low in mood or lacking energy, the use of a stimulant such as amphetamine or cocaine is perceived as a guaranteed way of feeling more alert and energised, at least in the short term. Many young people learn that alcohol, for instance, can aid social interaction, making it easier to fit in when taking part in social activities. The reality is that many social occasions available to young people are associated with the use of alcohol, illicit drugs or both. Young people also use substances to help them deal with emotional difficulties, which may be especially appealing to someone who might have numerous problems in their life, or who may already be experiencing mental distress. Using substances may help to alter the perception of their problems in the short term. Some young people become habitual users of substances, resulting in physical or psychological withdrawal if they attempt to cut down or quit their current usage.

CANNABIS AND MENTAL HEALTH

Cannabis is the most widely used illicit drug consumed by young people in the UK, and among those attending early intervention mental health services. The potential link between its usage and the onset and course of mental health problems has been debated in several studies.[14-16] These studies have suggested a causal link between the use of cannabis, especially if started at an early age, and the subsequent development of psychosis. There is now evidence that cannabis may play an important role in the development of psychotic illness in high-risk groups.[14] There appears to be an increased risk of any psychotic outcome in individuals who had ever used cannabis.[17] Professionals working in early intervention mental health teams need a functional knowledge of cannabis and how it affects mental health. It is also useful to have an understanding of the types of cannabis that individuals are using and the patterns of use. Professionals need to have informed conversations with the individual about cannabis in an honest and open fashion.

KEY POINT 6.3

There are many different types of cannabis, all of which have different strengths.

Knowing what type of cannabis and how much a person is using can be helpful to pinpoint early signs of relapse. This could be related to an increase in cannabis use or a change in type of cannabis to a stronger variety. Professionals in early intervention services need to have knowledge about cannabis that is readily accessible and up to date. The UK government's own drugs advisory service – Talk to Frank – provides good and non-judgemental information: www.talktofrank.com (accessed 17 January 2011).

REFLECTIVE PRACTICE EXERCISE 6.1

Time: 20 minutes
Consider a young person you know – either a person you have worked alongside or someone you have got to know outside of work – a friend, neighbour or acquaintance.

Without the opportunity to sit down and ask them, how much do you know about their lifestyle choices around drink, prescribed and/or illicit substance use?

Until you are able to have a conversation with them about this matter, how confident are you that you are able to understand the reasons why they drink or use other substances?

ADDRESSING MENTAL HEALTH–SUBSTANCE USE NEEDS

The effects of mental health–substance use problems may cause ongoing distress and disruption. They may also be a major factor in continuing to use or in returning to use substances, especially if the person believes that they are playing a role. Substance use professionals often find this frustrating, and the individual may find it self-defeating, leading to pessimistic prognoses on both sides. Professionals may not feel confident in detecting and assessing mental health problems. When they are able to identify them, they may be at a loss to address them. They might not have the skills needed to offer mental health interventions or the knowledge of services to know how or where to refer. Attitudes and values concerning mental ill health may not reflect the kind of non-judgemental or empathic understanding that is helpful in ensuring optimistic outcomes.

If services are aiming to improve engagement and clinical outcomes for individuals experiencing mental health–substance use problems, they need to focus their efforts on improving training of professionals, providing robust supervision structures and improving joint-working initiatives among agencies. All of these issues are especially important when addressing the needs of young people entering early intervention services, as professionals will meet many young people experiencing mental health–substance use issues. Professionals need empowerment in offering advice and individualised interventions for mental health–substance use problems.

The use of illicit drugs among young people with a vulnerability to psychosis appears to be a potentially dangerous behaviour and appears to supersede the dangers of drinking alcohol alone. Drug use without alcohol use has been associated with a highly significant increase in days spent in hospital.[18] There may be a 'supersensitivity' to even quite small amounts of the drug.[19] Families and carers of young people experiencing mental health–substance use problems often report that they had noticed changes in a young person's thoughts, feelings and behaviours at the time that illicit drug use had been noticed. This causes great concern to families and leads to arguments, bewilderment and despair. Families often reach the conclusion that substance use directly leads to mental health problems and that if the young person would stop using drugs, all the problems would disappear. However, this is often not the case.

EFFECTIVE INTERVENTIONS

A growing evidence base displays the effectiveness of comprehensive, integrated approaches that address mental health–substance use problems. 'Traditional' 12-step-style interventions, based on abstinence, were the first interventions to be investigated, with initially disappointing results.[20] It has been suggested that these early studies did not address the complexity of the individual's presenting problems.

Later research used comprehensive programmes that included assertive outreach. They also based the psychological interventions around the principles of health-behaviour change, using a motivational interviewing approach.[21]

Many studies that display the effectiveness of integrated treatments have been published.[22-30] These studies, although all different in design, participants, interventions and measured outcomes, used assertive outreach principles with a long-term perspective that offered stepwise interventions, motivational interviewing, education around drug use and its effect on mental health, and interventions in areas such as help with housing, finance and increased social support.

One of these studies[29,30] was carried out in the UK and is now being followed up by the Motivational Interventions for Drugs and Alcohol misuse in Schizophrenia (MIDAS) trial, a large multi-site randomised controlled trial into the efficacy of motivational interviewing and cognitive behavioural therapy.[31] This trial will be the largest study to date into the efficacy of comprehensive and integrated treatments.

DETECTING SUBSTANCE USE

Mental health professionals, especially those who work with vulnerable young people, must be able to detect and assess substance use. Effective detection and assessment can best be undertaken if the individual and professional are engaged honestly and openly. A non-judgemental attitude towards the young person and their lifestyle choices needs to be employed.

SELF-ASSESSMENT EXERCISE 6.2

Time: 20 minutes
- Consider your attitude towards a young person with these problems.
- What do you notice about yourself?

- How can you ensure that your own approach is non-judgemental?
- As human beings, can we be totally non-judgemental towards those within our care?
- Answer honestly and openly and acknowledge how hard this is.

Once this has been accomplished, the following questions must be addressed:
➤ Which substances are being used?
➤ How much is the individual using?
➤ How often are they using – for instance, are they using every day or just once or twice a week?
➤ Which method of drug use are they employing – are they smoking, swallowing, snorting or injecting?
➤ How long have they been doing so?
➤ How are they getting the money to buy substances?
➤ What are the effects of the substance used – both good and not so good?
➤ What, if anything, do they want to do about their drug use?

SELF-ASSESSMENT EXERCISE 6.3

Time: 10 minutes
What are the possible barriers to truth telling for the individual?

Although these would appear to be obvious questions to ask, it is surprising how often young people are either unwilling or unable to give accurate answers to them. The unwillingness is sometimes because of fears of stigma or fear of admitting to an illegal activity that may lead to problems with the police or exclusion from school or college. Inability to accurately measure their own substance use may be because of:
➤ the often chaotic nature of substance use
➤ the impairment that may accompany substance use
➤ lack of thought about the subject.

The use of drink and drug daily diaries can often be helpful in gaining a more accurate picture of the extent and circumstances of substance use.

REFLECTIVE PRACTICE EXERCISE 6.2

Time: 20 minutes
- Reflect back to the person you identified in Reflective Practice Exercise 6.1.
- What questions would you need to ask them to establish exactly what substances they are taking and what impact these substances have/had on their life?
- How confident would you be about asking these questions in a way that was acceptable to the young person and that provided you with the best chance to gain this information?

> • How comfortable would you be about asking these questions?
>
> These require you to think deeply about yourself and your own responses.

PRACTICAL WAYS OF EFFECTIVE WORKING

The evidence base for effective interventions for people experiencing mental health–substance use problems is becoming well established and is based on comprehensive, integrated approaches. To work effectively with young people who have first-onset psychosis and who are simultaneously continuing to use substances, professionals need to encourage and sustain a degree of therapeutic optimism.

KEY POINT 6.4

An acknowledgment of the uniqueness of the individual is important, as is a non-judgemental attitude.

Professionals should display empathy about the individual's present situation – and how the person arrived there. The development of engagement skills is especially important and professionals may have to employ a range of creative and opportunistic strategies when working with hard-to-engage young people around issues of substance use. Education and health promotion information must be delivered, not via a general formula but in an individual way to each person, based on the person's existing knowledge, and in a form and language that is acceptable to her/him.[32]

The most effective interventions aimed at young people experiencing mental health–substance use problems appear to be ones that are based on a genuine collaboration, addressing the individual's own priorities rather than those of the services. Effective interventions include conversations around health-behaviour change and taking time to establish where the individual is in terms of change, promoting a stepwise targeted approach, as opposed to a rigid formulation based on where the professional expects the person to be at, at any given time.

Professionals engaging young people need to be realistic about expecting these individuals to change the way they behave just because health professionals and their families believe that they should, or because they ought to do so. For families it may seem the sensible thing to do when helping the young person improve their mental health, or reduce the problems in their lives. However, young people, whether they have an early onset of psychosis or not, have individualised health-behaviour needs and expectations that may differ from those of health professionals and others who care about them. For many young people, their mental or physical health is not of high priority. They may believe that they are invulnerable or that the benefits of taking substances are currently outweighing the drawbacks. They may have decided that stopping their substance use or cutting down the amount they are using is not possible at the present time – even though they may decide to change their behaviours eventually. It appears that for some young people, interventions such as providing acceptable information about cannabis use may be worth considering before attempting more intensive therapeutic input.[33]

Case study 6.1: Alison

Background

Alison (24) describes a normal and happy childhood until she was about 14 years of age. She did well at school and was a popular and diligent pupil. She says that she had always got on well with her mum and dad and was always a 'good girl'. However, when she was 14 her parents separated and her father moved out of the family home. Alison found this upsetting and she started to have arguments with her mum. She also started to play truant from school and began to stay out at night. At around this time she started to drink alcohol with friends and also experimented with cannabis. She eventually left school with no qualifications and her relationship with her mum deteriorated further when she refused to return either to complete her education or to get a job. By the time she was 18, she was, in her own words, 'running wild'. She had become friendly with a group of other young people, none of whom were working or attending college. Her mum tried to restrict her behaviour and to influence her to do something with her life but this only caused increasingly acrimonious arguments between them.

By this time, Alison was also anxious and depressed. She began to cut her arms and the inside of her thighs as a way of relieving herself of some of her distressing feelings but this resulted in a further loss of her confidence and self-esteem. She also began to notice that when she smoked cannabis she became increasingly paranoid. She began to find it very difficult to be with other people in social situations. Using public transport was a particularly distressing experience. This made her want to do even less with her time, except to hang out with her friends, drinking and smoking cannabis. However, by this time she realised that cannabis made her distressed. Alison was reluctant to stop because it helped her to fit in with the other group members and it had become a routine part of her life.

Her mum eventually ran out of patience. After one especially difficult argument, her mum told her to pack her bags and leave. Alison ended up sleeping in friends' houses when she could ('sofa surf'). She never actually had to sleep on the street but she came quite close to it on occasions. Her mental health deteriorated even further during this period and after a more serious incident of self-harm (an overdose of paracetamol tablets following a row with her boyfriend) she ended up in her local emergency department. Alison was referred to the mental health service for assessment. The professional concluded that she might have the beginning of a psychotic illness and referred her to the local 'early intervention for psychosis' service.

The early intervention team provided a full psychosocial assessment. This resulted in Alison being accepted by the service, and over the next six months she received help in a range of areas. A place was found for her in a specialist support hostel for young people with mental health problems and she was given help with accessing appropriate benefits. She was prescribed a trial dose of antipsychotic medication and some of her distressing symptoms began to diminish. However, she continued to smoke cannabis on a regular basis, although it still made her paranoid.

Interventions around substance use (based on Bodkin, *et al.*[13])

Although most of the professionals in the early intervention team thought that it would be of great benefit to Alison's mental health for her to give up cannabis use, it was important to them to remain neutral and non-judgemental towards her when discussing this issue. However, this did not stop them from taking her cannabis use seriously and keeping the subject on the agenda during conversations with her. They also made sure to check whether she was taking other drugs and discovered that, apart from occasional alcohol use, she was not taking any other substances. Alison confided that her decision to cut down her alcohol use was because she had been putting on lots of weight and she had heard that alcohol was full of calories. Alison had not found it difficult to cut down her alcohol use because she had never enjoyed the effects of it very much. However, she reported that at present she did not want to change her current cannabis use, although she acknowledged that this was something she might eventually consider. It was the early intervention service's usual practice to involve family members in all aspects of care. However, Alison was still almost entirely estranged from both her parents at this time, so this was not possible.

The next important step in intervention was to provide education on the psychological risks of cannabis use. Information about cannabis and its potential effects on mental state was provided. Before this was given, the professional clearly established Alison's existing knowledge and understanding about cannabis and mental health, and how she interpreted this information. This helped the professional to understand clearly what Alison already knew about cannabis, and elicited her views about the part it played in her life, and what, if anything, she wished to change. Permission was obtained to supplement this information with individualised, accessible and acceptable information in the form of a booklet and a brief DVD presentation. At the next session, the professional was then able to discuss with Alison what she thought of the new information and what she wanted to do with it.

Alison and the professional had, by this time, developed a collaborative relationship based on honesty and trust. This enabled them to discuss, for the first time in Alison's life, the reasons for her cannabis use, which included fitting in with her peers, helping her to relax and to relieve the boredom and tedium that she experienced due to her lack of worthwhile and stimulating activity. This conversation enabled them to generate alternative strategies to gain the same benefits without the use of cannabis. Alison confided that one of the things that prevented her from attempting to cut down or quit her cannabis use was a lack of confidence in her ability to do so. The professional reminded Alison that she had been able to reduce her use of alcohol and that she seemed to be a resourceful person who could make and sustain significant changes when she decided to do so.

Alison still smokes cannabis. She is considering cutting down and has begun to acknowledge that she wants to quit altogether sometime in the future. It remains an important agenda item on her care plan and Alison and the team regularly discuss her current cannabis use.

REFLECTIVE PRACTICE EXERCISE 6.3

Time: 20 minutes
- Does the approach adopted by Alison's early intervention services fit in with your current way of working with people who use substances problematically?
- What are the advantages of this approach?
- Is there anything about this approach that makes you feel uncomfortable or uneasy? If so, what and why?

CONCLUSION

KEY POINT 6.5

Substance use remains common in young people.

Young people with a vulnerability to psychotic symptoms are no different from others. The pessimism that has accompanied these individuals in the past is beginning to be challenged by a growing evidence base that refutes these attitudes. Professionals are beginning to understand how to engage individuals in a range of interventions that address mental health–substance use needs and it is important that families and carers are supported to cope with the distress these issues can cause. Flexible and timely services can work with young people who continue to use drink and drugs, even when this behaviour appears to be adversely affecting their mental health. Young people take substances for a variety of reasons, for example:
- they believe that they help to relieve symptoms
- they think that they reduce some of the side effects of medication
- they sometimes offer a quick way to feel a little better or to relieve boredom
- they are an area of their lives that they feel they still have some *control* over
- they would prefer to be labelled a 'drug user' than someone with a 'mental health problem'
- substances are cheap, freely available and can be very enjoyable.

A collaborative and non-judgemental approach towards individuals enables the professional to display empathy, avoid confrontation and support self-efficacy. This can enhance the process of engagement and can lead to some individuals choosing to make sustained changes that can play an important part in their recovery from psychosis.

REFERENCES

1 Regier D, Farmer M, Rae D, et al. Comorbidity of mental disorders with alcohol and other drugs of abuse: results from the epidemiological catchment area (ECA) study. *Journal of the American Medical Association.* 1990; **264**: 2511–8.

2 Gibbins J, Kipping C. Coexistent substance use and psychiatric disorders. In: Gamble C, Brennan G, editors. *Working with Serious Mental Illness.* Edinburgh: Elsevier; 2006.

3 Menezes P, Johnson S, Thornicroft G, et al. Drug and alcohol problems among people with severe mental illness in South London. *British Journal of Psychiatry.* 1996; **168**: 612–9.

4 Duke PJ, Pantelis C, Barnes TR. South Westminster schizophrenia survey: alcohol use and its relationship to symptoms, tardive dyskinesia and illness onset. *British Journal of Psychiatry.* 1994; **164**: 630–6.

5 Green B, Young R, Kavanagh D. Cannabis use and misuse prevalence among people with psychosis. *British Journal of Psychiatry.* 2005; **187**: 306–13.

6 Banerjee S, Clancy C, Crome I. *Co-existing Problems of Mental Disorder and Substance Misuse (Dual Diagnosis): an information manual.* London: Royal College of Psychiatrists Research Unit; 2002.

7 Weaver T, Renton A, Stimson G, et al. Comorbidity of substance misuse and mental illness in community mental health and substance misuse. *British Journal of Psychiatry.* 2003; **183**: 304–13.

8 Cantwell R, Brewin J, Glazebrook C, et al. Prevalence of substance use in first-episode psychosis. *British Journal of Psychiatry.* 1999; **174**: 150–3.

9 Barnett JH, Werners U, Secher SM, et al. Substance use in a population-based clinic sample of people with first-episode psychosis. *British Journal of Psychiatry.* 2007; **190**: 515–20.

10 Costa e Silva JA. Evidence-based analysis of the worldwide abuse of licit and illicit drugs. *Human Psychopharmacology.* 2002; **17**: 131–40.

11 Hoare J. *Drug Misuse Declared: findings from the 2008/09 British crime survey, England and Wales* [Home Office Statistical Bulletin]. London: The Home Office; 2009.

12 European Monitoring Centre for Drug & Drug Addiction. *2001 Annual Report on the State of the Drugs Problem in the European Union.* Brussels: European Monitoring Centre for Drug & Drug Addiction; 2001.

13 Bodkin LL, Singh A, Corcoran C. Cannabis as a risk factor for psychosis in vulnerable teens: implications for treatment. *Primary Psychiatry.* 2008; **15**: 51–7.

14 Arseneault L, Cannon M, Poulton R, et al. Cannabis use in adolescence and risk for adult psychosis: longitudinal prospective study. *British Medical Journal.* 2002; **325**: 1212–3.

15 Van Os J, Hanssen M, Bijl RV, et al. Cannabis use and psychosis: a longitudinal population study. *American Journal of Epidemiology.* 2002; **156**: 319–27.

16 Zammit S, Allebeck P, Andreasson S, et al. Self-reported cannabis use as a risk factor for schizophrenia in Swedish conscripts of 1969: historical cohort study. *British Medical Journal.* 2002; **325**: 1199.

17 Moore TH, Zammit S, Lingford-Hughes A, et al. Cannabis use and risk of psychotic or affective mental health outcomes: a systematic review. *Lancet.* 2007; **370**: 319–28.

18 Crebbin K, Mitford E, Paxton R, et al. Drug and alcohol misuse in first episode psychosis: an observational study. *Neuropsychiatric Disease and Treatment.* 2008; **4**: 417–23.

19 Mueser K, Bennett M, Kushner MG. Epidemiology of substance use disorders among persons with chronic mental illness. In: Lehman A, Dixon L, editors. *Double Jeopardy: chronic mental illness and substance use disorders.* Switzerland: Harwood Academic; 1995.

20 Ley A, Jeffery DP, McClaren S, et al. Treatment programmes for people with both severe mental illness and substance misuse. *Cochrane Database Syst Rev.* 2000; 2:CD001088.

21 Miller W, Rollnick S. *Motivational Interviewing: preparing people to change addictive behaviour*. New York: Guilford Press; 2002.
22 Godley SH, Hoewing-Roberson R, Godley MD. *Final MISA Report*. Bloomington Illinois: Lighthouse; 1994.
23 Jerrell JM, Ridgely MS. Comparative effectiveness of three approaches to serving people with severe mental illness and substance use disorders. *Journal of Nervous and Mental Disease*. 1995; **183**: 566–76.
24 Drake R, Yovetich NA, Bebout RR, *et al*. Integrated treatment for dually diagnosed homeless adults. *Journal of Nervous and Mental Disease*. 1997; **185**: 298–305.
25 Carmichael D. *Texas DD Project Evaluation Report, 1997–1998*. College Station, Texas: A&M University Public Policy Research Unit; 1998.
26 Drake RE, McHugo GJ, Clark RE, *et al*. Assertive community treatment for patients with co-occurring severe mental illness and substance use disorder: a clinical trial. *American Journal of Orthopsychiatry*. 1998; **68**: 201–15.
27 Ho AP, Tsuang JW, Liberman RP. Achieving effective treatment of patients with chronic psychotic illness and comorbid substance dependence. *American Journal of Psychiatry*. 1999; **156**: 1765–70.
28 Brunette MF, Drake RE, Woods M, *et al*. A comparison of long-term and short-term residential treatment programmes for dual diagnosis patients. *Psychiatric Services*. 2001; **52**: 526–8.
29 Barrowclough C, Haddock G, Tarrier N, *et al*. Randomized controlled trial of motivational interviewing, cognitive behaviour therapy, and family intervention for patients with comorbid schizophrenia and substance use disorders. *American Journal of Psychiatry*. 2001; **158**: 1706–13.
30 Haddock G, Barrowclough C, Tarrier N, *et al*. Cognitive behavioural therapy and motivational intervention for schizophrenia and substance misuse: 18-month outcomes of a randomised controlled trial. *British Journal of Psychiatry*. 2003; **183**: 418–26.
31 Barrowclough C, Haddock G, Lowens I, *et al*. Psychosis and drug and alcohol problems. In: Baker A, Velleman R, editors. *A Clinical Handbook of Co-existing Mental Health and Drug and Alcohol Problems*. London: Routledge; 2007.
32 Butters JE. The impact of peers and social disapproval on high-risk cannabis use: gender differences and implications for drug education. *Drugs: Education, Prevention and Policy*. 2004; **11**: 381–90.
33 Edwards JK, Elkins K, Hinton M, *et al*. Randomized controlled trial of a cannabis-focused intervention for young people with first-episode psychosis. *Acta Psychiatrica Scandinavica*. 2006; **114**: 109–17.

TO LEARN MORE

- Information about cannabis and mental health from the Royal College of Psychiatrists – available at: www.rcpsych.ac.uk/mentalhealthinfo/youngpeople/cannabis.aspx (accessed 7 February 2011)
- Government sites:
  www.drugs.gov.uk (accessed 17 January 2011).
  www.talktofrank.com (accessed 17 January 2011).

CHAPTER 7

Engaging the individual and family

David Watkins, Francis McCormick and Rosemary Cuff

PRE-READING EXERCISE 7.1

Time: 45 minutes

Think about the Browns, a family of five with mid-range socioeconomic standing, who live in the urban environment of a city with a population of 1.2 million people. The father, Paul, is an accountant with a commercial sales firm. He comes from a middle-class family and is an only child. His wife, Margaret, stays at home and provides the major homemaker role. Their three children, Emily, Sean and Michael, aged 16, 14 and 10, attend a local secondary school. They have been returning mixed scholastic results, although their abilities are strong.

Margaret suffers from depression and is a binge alcohol user. She has suffered from recurrent episodes of depression since her early 20s and she is reluctant to use antidepressant medication as she feels it makes her tired, and this affects her ability as a wife and mother. Significantly, the tiredness also interferes with her personal interests outside the family, which has always been important to her for her sense of individuality.

Paul and Margaret often argue in front of the children when Margaret is drunk. She tends to binge 2–3 times a week, to the point of intoxication. She tends to be confrontational and unreasonable at these times. Paul has always had a tendency to be dismissive of Margaret when she raises issues of parenting with him. Paul deals with disagreements with Margaret by threatening to leave her if she does not stop drinking. Emily and Sean feel that they need to 'umpire' the disagreement between their parents. This causes them to take sides at times and defend the parent they feel is aggrieved, although they don't always take the same side! Michael, the youngest, is confused by the problems within the family and, as a result, tends to remove himself from the scene of the dispute and withdraw to his room to play computer games.

Consider the Browns and their situation:

1 What are some of the issues or concerns from the perspective of each individual family member?
2 What are some of the issues that may be confronting the family as a unit?
3 List five potential issues (both professional/service system and family-based) that may hinder successful engagement in services for this family.

4   How may these be overcome by a mental health–substance use professional?

Write your answers down.

INTRODUCTION

This chapter looks at the impact of mental health–substance use upon family life and will help the reader consider and reflect upon some of the important roles that a family plays. It discusses particular ways the mental health–substance use professional may engage and work with families living with mental health–substance use problems, including how their relationship with the individual helps with family engagement. Finally, it examines how service systems may be used as a tool to cause effective and sustainable change.

VALUING THE ROLES OF THE FAMILY

In Western sociological terms, families are made up of individuals who form themselves into a unique and integrated functional social system. The goals of a family are varied depending upon the individual perspective, but generally include the socialisation and enculturation of members, procreation, meeting attachment, developmental and emotional needs, and may also serve political and religious ends. The authors take a broad approach to the definition of a family in this chapter. What may be said is that we view families as having differing members and structures, and in a general sense having common purposes and sets of conventions and customs based upon the experiences of their members.

REFLECTIVE PRACTICE EXERCISE 7.1

Time: 45 minutes
Spend some time thinking about your own experiences of 'family life'. Reflect on your views and ask yourself what might be the factors that shape your views. Things to think about include:
- membership or composition
- relationships
- communication
- cultural factors
- religious factors
- migration
- extended family
- proximity
- generational values.

Consider your definition of family and how your experience of family may influence your choice of career and perception of working with families. Specifically, are there key aspects that motivate you to seek or avoid performing family-based work? Write your thoughts down.

Evidence suggests that the family can play an important protective role in the life of someone with mental health and/or substance use problems;[1,2] a loving family that offers unconditional acceptance is central to a family supporting one of its own. However, family members and home life can also play an adverse role that perpetuates long-term substance use if, for example, the background familial factors are themselves negative.[3]

Many people who experience mental illness and substance use disorders, by the time they are linked with services, have disconnected from or have tenuous relationships with their family. Nonetheless, despite seemingly having 'no family' involvement, they and the family always have a relationship regardless of the level of contact, and can wish for actual improvement or at least personal resolution. Recognising and understanding a person's motivations for seeking help may help to provide information about their relationship with their family and any underlying familial factors that may have influenced them to seek help; for men, the reason that they seek treatment may be because of their family or carer insisting that they do so.[4] Effective engagement with both the individual and their family may also help to restore relationships that have been damaged through mental health–substance use problems.

REFLECTIVE PRACTICE EXERCISE 7.2

Time: 40 minutes

Earlier you thought about your views on 'family life' and wrote down some of the factors that shape those views. Now think about how these views may influence mental health–substance use problems if they occurred within your 'context' or family. In two columns, one labelled Protecting Factors and one labelled Perpetuating Factors, make a list of your thoughts.

MENTAL HEALTH–SUBSTANCE USE AND FAMILY LIFE

Parents who experience mental health–substance use issues can face challenges such as isolation, poverty, higher rates of family violence and offending, and community stigma (*see* Book 1, Chapters 4, 7 and 8).[5] The cumulative effect on children and young people can increase risk factors such as developmental delay, school refusal and significant behavioural issues.[6] Children take on caring responsibilities – ranging from domestic chores to emotional care and nursing-type tasks – when there is no one else available to care.[7] The carer burden can indeed be high for both the younger and older carer.

The family may have little understanding of the interaction between mental health issues and a substance use problem. Mueser and Fox[8] looked at a summary of families' needs based on several published works. The needs they found were for information about comorbid disorders, and tools to help minimise familial stress and to provide assistance with problem-solving. It follows, then, that families are naturally placed to contribute to recovery of the person. Typically, though, each member of the family may have a differing need or a differing priority of needs. Some may be seeking information for themselves; some may be seeking information for others; or they may have a principal aim to provide some form of practical, psychological or emotional support. All are equally important objectives. Identifying the different needs of family members is an early and important task to accomplish. This should be developed over time to allow the family's trust and confidence to develop in the professional, without forcing the family members to change their sequence of operation,[9] but allowing them to adapt and change in their own time phases and cycles. Although it may take time for trust to develop, this process can be enhanced by the professional's approach and qualities such as openness and respect.

If there appears to be little progress over time with getting the family members to identify their needs, analysing this with Prochaska and colleagues'[10] Model for Change (*see* Book 4, Chapter 6) may reflect how a family is positioned in relation to their family member's mental health–substance use problem. This model, which describes a cyclical model of substance use and recovery, can provide a structure to understand the varying phases of the individual's pattern of use and behaviour. In these cases, the use of this model as both an assessment and an intervention tool can be useful. For example, in the Brown family, Mr Brown can be viewed as being in the action phase, whereas Mrs Brown is in the precontemplative stage. Insights of this type can guide the professional and may also be useful in helping to develop a psycho-education approach with the family.

Some tools can greatly enhance family practice work. A personal and family care plan (*see* Box 7.1) can be a very important and practical tool to help clarify and document family needs and wishes.[11] Family care plans (FCPs) can promote thoughtful and considered input by all parties, particularly when the individual is in good health, so that their wishes are clear in times when they may relapse or be less able to advocate for themselves. FCPs are an essential part of a therapeutic intervention (*see* Book 4, Chapter 2) when there are dependent children in the family. They help to identify relapse warning signs, preferred outcomes for all family members, and the people who can be contacted for help when things are not going to plan.[11] Identifying both crisis and care components are necessary inclusions for FCPs, such as future planning for possible crises and longer-term goals – for example, children's education plans.

BOX 7.1 Personal and family care plan

Example personal care plan
Check with Mum and Dad about making this plan and that they agree with it when it is finished.

Fill this out as best as you can, print it out and then put it somewhere safe where you can find it.

Somewhere I can go when things get scary is:
A person I trust who could help if I'm in a situation that worries me is:
Their phone number is:
Things I can do to help me get less stressed are (e.g. go to my room to play, phone a friend, listen to music, talk to someone):

a

b

c

d

e

Now that you have made your Personal Care Plan, be sure to print it out and put it somewhere safe where you can find it.

Example family care plan
Important phone numbers
The mental health team phone number is:
My parents' case manager/workers' name is:
Their phone number is:

Two other adults I can call:
Name:
Phone Number:
Name:
Phone Number:

I know my Mum/Dad is getting unwell when I notice:

Now that you have made your family care plan, be sure to print it out and put it somewhere safe where you can find it.

The first contact with the family or an individual carer may be born from crisis. Mueser and Fox[8] described illness relapses, substance bingeing, violence and loss of accommodation as examples of these crises. At these times, the family's main requirement may be to seek a resolution of the crisis and, as such, is an opportunity for them to be heard. A crisis can also be viewed as an opportunity for change and for the individual and family to re-evaluate their circumstances.[12] Therefore, at these times a problem-solving and solution focused orientation will provide the most successful connection with them (*see* Chapter 10; Book 4, Chapter 7). Care does need to be taken when providing support for decisions at the moment of crisis. Professional judgement may be required to support and encourage the motivation to change, or, conversely, advise caution with hasty decisions or plans. For example, considering the Brown family from earlier in the chapter, Mrs Brown may, after a binge, be motivated to seek assistance, although possible guilt about the impact on the children could encourage either change or further decline if she feels defeated, or that it is too late to change.

REFLECTIVE PRACTICE EXERCISE 7.3

Time: 30 minutes
What would be helpful to Mrs Brown to encourage her to seek assistance after a binge?

- How could the family help her?
- What barriers may be in her way?
- How could you, as the professional working alongside Mrs Brown, help facilitate change?

ENGAGING FAMILIES: THE PRACTICE CONTEXT
Determining the circumstances of the family

It must be remembered that a one-size-fits-all approach to a family is, more than likely, doomed to fail. There are too many competing dimensions when mental health–substance use problems are present, including stage of recovery, diagnoses, level of functioning, impact of the problem, degree of acuteness, motivation, personal predisposition, and readiness and capacity to access the service system. Therefore, providing a comprehensive assessment and a formulation based on needs, coupled with a flexible approach, is most likely to afford the greatest benefit for all.

Providing a full and comprehensive assessment of the family need and function is, therefore, vital. This assessment should include family strengths as well as any difficulties. This can be developed with gentle curiosity around the usual routine, 'house rules', previous handling of difficult situations and support and their culture. Prefacing this task with the purpose of your enquiry aids engagement, and the accuracy of the information gained. In addition, it is important to directly assess children and young person's need with their developmental progress in mind and not to assume they will understand the process of assessment or automatically engage with it.

Engaging the family

Gaining consent to include the family in the work with the individual is, of course, paramount. Some individuals may be very reluctant to give consent to speak to the family if they have not addressed problems with them previously. If an organisation and its professionals have an expectation and understanding about what a desired level of family involvement is, as well as what the focus of this involvement will be,[13] making this known should encourage family contact. Having clear organisational expectations gives the professional clarity and the confidence to explain the benefits for family involvement to the individual and their family, thus improving engagement.

When first engaging a family, introduce an expectation of change while also validating previous attempts. This will help you when the individual and their family or carer may be at quite different stages of need. It reflects that, even if they are at different stages, they share a common element together. The most important task at this time is for the professional to try to synchronise these needs so that the family or carer may be in the best position to assist the individual, while simultaneously having their own needs met. At this time, information and support to the family or carer is critical. Sometimes, however, the family might overtake the individual in the treatment cycle. If this happens, the professional needs to temper the expectations of the family or carer so that they do not exceed those of the individual.

In recent years, there has been a greater involvement of families and carers in mental health–substance use services. However, relatively speaking, this is still a fairly recent phenomena and some families and carers may not be used to being involved in the treatment process. Some may have trepidation or wariness about becoming involved because of previous experiences. Box 7.2 offers the top ten tips for family engagement.

BOX 7.2 Top ten tips for family engagement

1   Be socially engaging with each person. Have conversations with the family to get to know them. From first meeting, advertise that you are open and expect contact with family members.

2   Look for opportunistic contact. For example, walk out with the individual if the family are waiting outside the office, at least to introduce yourself.

3   Develop rules of communication. Model transparency and negotiate agreement on confidentiality. Seek mutual understanding on how and what information is shared, and what is reasonable to be kept private to the individual.

4   Set up 'special meetings'. Use an agenda or meeting structure to assist the interview with families. Professionals new to the field of family work have usually had some experience in participating in groups or facilitating 'meetings' and can transfer these skills to a new context.

5   Use genograms (family tree/constellations) to promote conversation as well as for practical documentation.

6   Talk about the tough things as these issues are usually on the individual's and family's minds. For example, acknowledge possible blame and frustration and be mindful of non-verbal interactions. Promote discussion and clarify and validate the experience, but be cautious of exacerbating blame or other unhelpful processes.

7   Provide relevant no-nonsense information that is accurate and concise. Be prepared to go over information at another time – in stressful moments some important information may not be fully understood. Avoid jargon and acronyms. Providing written information (in a native tongue) can be beneficial.

8   Build the relationship and trust. Provide practical assistance if appropriate, or initiate contact in non-crisis times, as this may enhance collaboration especially in difficult times.

9   Constantly review and reflect with the individual and family to promote mutual agreement on goals and approach to working together. Include the family in care planning; revisit plans, especially if there was initial refusal to have the family involved.

10 Be consistent, doing what you say you will do, and being clear if you are unable to do it. Apologise if need be.

REFLECTIVE PRACTICE EXERCISE 7.4

Time: 30 minutes
- Suggest five of your own best practice tips. Write them down for later reference.

Working with younger family members of the individual

Often the role of the professional can be as 'coach' for the parent to assist them (or co-facilitate family discussion) with explaining and supporting their children/family member. At other times, the professional may work more directly with a young person. The young person needs to be aware that parents have given permission and agreed on how information will be shared or remain confidential. The professional needs to work in a developmentally appropriate framework to ensure that they are explaining the problem in a way that the younger person understands. It is important to reassure them that the problem may not happen to them, nor is it their fault, as well as assist them to understand their feelings about what is happening around them. Teenage males in particular may have difficulty talking about their problems. Stanhope and colleagues[14] recommended initially talking about a broad range of subjects to help to gain the confidence of the person. Westwood and Pinzon[15] also support this type of approach.

Grief for a young person can be heightened in families and their carers may accept behaviours or symptoms associated with grief as a 'phase', thus delaying proactive action or treatment. Therefore, rapport development with the younger family members is important. After initial rapport building, some of the areas that you might consider talking to younger people about include:
- what to do in an emergency
- taking care of yourself
- looking out for brothers and sisters
- where to turn to for further help
- educational needs around mental health problems and issues
- sense of burden
- maintaining hope
- acknowledging the disruption to their life.

REFLECTIVE PRACTICE EXERCISE 7.5

Time: 15 minutes
Write down four more examples of issues you may raise with a younger family member of an individual.

Finally, avoid engagement barriers such as offering only office-based appointment approaches. Use flexible patterns of service provision such as shorter appointments, and use text messaging, email or social networking sites to contact younger people with prompts and reminders of appointments – but only where privacy and confidentiality can be assured.

Remember, an important question to consider is: 'Is it that the family/individual is not ready for assistance or has the professional/organisation not yet found a way to engage?'

Working with families that appear reluctant to engage (or 'hard-to-engage' families)

It is generally acknowledged that service engagement by individuals can be problematic within both the mental health and the substance use treatment sectors. However, is this non-compliance or is it choice? The reasons for poor engagement are varied and complex.[16] When maintenance of engagement is at risk, Mueser and Fox[8] have suggested that active service involvement may lead to a better outcome for the ongoing relationship between the individual and the service; for example, by providing practical assistance such as transportation, if that is what is required. It has been found that acts of kindness, pleasant surroundings and providing a desirable benefit promoted service use. In addition, the authors identify that the characteristics of the professional can be a factor. These include a more understanding attitude and a non-judgemental approach, and providing flexible availability on a walk-in basis, or in locations and at times that support and suit the young person.[17]

Be helpful! However, and this is a most important point, avoid making promises that cannot be kept. Woolfall and colleagues[18] found in their evaluation of Families First (an intensive family intervention programme) that people felt it was preferable to be not promised anything at all rather than experience loss of trust if something that was promised was not delivered. Start small and build up to bigger outcomes.

Using yourself and the individual relationship as a means of engagement

Much like a tradesperson, a good professional needs to have a kit of quality tools to work effectively. These tools need to be honed regularly and kept ready for use when the time comes. In all settings, the universal tool at the ready disposal of the professional is one's self and one's alliance with the individual, or, as Wolfe and Goldfried[19] have described it, the *'quintessential integrative variable'*. While the research tends to point towards the therapeutic alliance as having a positive effect on the engagement and retention of people in substance use treatment, the intrinsic factors that determine this alliance are less well understood.[20] Nonetheless, this relationship forms the basis for therapeutic interventions, as well as being a framework for enabling positive outcomes for the work itself.[21]

Professional skills need to be built on this concept so that they can be effective in facilitating change and growth for people experiencing mental health–substance use problems. Critically, a good relationship with the individual and family will help to engage the individual and family in the therapeutic process. The professional's understanding of what is family work, or family-sensitive practice, may greatly influence their actual practice and willingness to be involved in family-inclusive work. *'Family sensitive practice can be considered as any work role that is performed in a way that is inclusive, understanding and respectful to families and other carers.'*[22]

Similarly, the level of confidence in addressing family issues will influence professional practice.[23] Family work can be viewed on a continuum, from practice that is loosely mindful of the family context (in one-to-one work alongside the identified individual), to comprehensive and expert family therapy and family-sensitive organisational structures. For the beginning professional, simple but powerful respectful practices can be helpful in promoting family engagement; for example, considering the impact on other family members when making service decisions, and validating and acknowledging the individual's concern for their family.

TABLE 7.1 Service principles and personal attributes

Service principle	Personal attribute
Looking to the evidence	Trust
An integrated approach to care and treatment	Commitment
Commitment	Knowledge, personal views and skills
Partnerships	Effective communication
A strengths-based approach	Trust in yourself
A non-assumptive approach	Empathy
Family-focused policy statements	Acceptance
Collaborative practice	Respect
Family-focused documentation	Positivism/hope

REFLECTIVE PRACTICE EXERCISE 7.6

Time: 60 minutes

There are several core principles and values the professional should draw upon to provide good clinical care and quality responses to individuals and their families. Think about the service principles and personal attributes in Table 7.1.

Rearrange them into an order that seems right to you.

- Which ones do you have; can you add more to the list?
- Which do you think you need to develop further?
- Why are these attributes and principles important to you?
- What principles as an organisation would you like to have at your work place?

Using the service system to foster family engagement

It may be generally said that there is a divide between mental health services and substance use services. The disorders are considered separately, rather than contemporaneously, though, in reality, this is far from the truth. This perception limits the response of both services to people experiencing mental health–substance use problems, and it also serves to distance the individual's family from the point of care. The inherent problem with this is described by O'Grady and Skinner,[24] who understand that there is a profound result of having a family member affected, and that there is strong desire to be educated on mental health–substance use problems as well as being involved throughout the treatment and recovery process.

Families in which mental health–substance use problems occur encounter a range of complex and often interrelated needs; it is not uncommon to find a range of government and non-government services involved with the same families. It has been recognised for some time that it is essential for services to work in a cohesive and coherent manner so that work is delivered in a coordinated fashion.[25]

Individuals within the family unit may be affected to differing degrees depending on their endowment, age and predisposition. They will have a variety of 'lenses' through which they view services, which may impact on their capacity to accept, advocate for or ask for support as they may have had negative experiences of service provision.

Service engagement can be enhanced by supportive relationships,[26] and a person-centred treatment approach can address the complex psychosocial dimensions of need, particularly working closely with, and in the context of, an individual's own social networks and family.[27]

Appropriate organisational policy and procedures that provide support and clarity to professionals, individuals and their families help build confidence in all parties. Family members and carers can provide a valuable and unique perspective and having them involved in the planning and delivery of services may be a positive step forward in developing quality practices. Another means by which this could be achieved is by providing family-centred waiting rooms, where toys, activities or books can occupy children and all feel welcomed.

REFLECTIVE PRACTICE EXERCISE 7.7

Time: 60 minutes
- To what extent do the policy and procedures in your organisation:
  - support the professional?
  - support the individual?
  - support the family?
- What changes could you suggest to modify or improve your organisation's policy and procedures?
- What would the Browns experience with your service? (Even if their circumstances did not meet the criteria for service, how would they receive re-referral?)

CONCLUSION

This chapter aimed to help the reader to consider and reflect upon some of the important roles that a family plays, and discussed how mental health–substance use problems can affect family life. It identified how a professional can help to strengthen family support systems, and enhance the outcomes for the person with a mental health–substance use problem.

This led to a discussion of particular ways the mental health–substance use professional may engage and work with families living with mental health–substance use problems. The professional can assist family members through support, education and explanation, particularly in families where there are young children. The exercises and examples in the chapter should help to guide and shape the reader's understanding and confidence in applying the practice principles described herein.

POST-READING EXERCISE 7.1

Time: 60 minutes

Think back to the Brown family who were introduced in Pre-reading Exercise 7.1. Now that you've had the opportunity to work through this chapter, reconsider these questions:

- What are some of the issues or concerns from the perspective of each individual family member?
- What are some of the issues that may be confronting the family as a unit?

Write your answers down and compare them with your earlier answers.

- How different do your answers now look when compared with your answers from Pre-reading Exercise 7.1?
- In what way are your answers different?
  - Have you developed a more conceptual framework of understanding of the value of family engagement?
  - Have you developed a greater practical understanding of some of the issues involved in working with the family of a person with mental health–substance use problems?
  - Has your attitude changed in the way you think about the importance of the family as an ally in a treatment strategy?
  - Do you think you would feel more confident in engaging the family in a treatment alliance?
  - How much do you think your skills may benefit from applying some of the approaches outlined in this chapter?

Re-examine your answers from Reflective Practice Exercises 7.4 and 7.5.

- Have your five best practice tips changed at all?
- Have you identified additional issues you may raise with a younger family member of an individual?

REFERENCES

1 Challier B, Chau N, Prédine R, *et al.* Associations of family environment and individual factors with tobacco, alcohol, and illicit drug use in adolescents. *European Journal of Epidemiology.* 2000; **16**: 33–42.

2 Johnson RA, Hoffman JP, Gerstein DR. *The Relationship Between Family Structure and Adolescent Substance Use.* Maryland: Substance Abuse and Mental Health Service Administration: Office of Applied Studies. US Department of Health and Human Services, Public Health Service; 1996.

3 Alverson H, Alverson M, Drake RE. An ethnographic study of the longitudinal course

of substance abuse among people with severe mental illness. *Community Mental Health Journal.* 2000; **36**: 557–69.

4 Watkins KE, Shaner A, Sullivan G. The role of gender in engaging the dually diagnosed in treatment. *Community Mental Health Journal.* 1999; **35**: 115–26.

5 Hegarty M. Supporting children affected by parental dual diagnosis – mental illness and substance use: a collaborative mental health promotion, prevention and early intervention initiative. *Auseinetter.* 2005; **25**: 21–6.

6 Finkelstein N, Rechberger E, Russell LA, *et al.* Building resilience in children of mothers who have co-occurring disorders and histories of violence: intervention model and implementation issues. *Journal of Behavioral Health Services and Research.* 2005; **32**: 141–54.

7 Aldridge J, Becker S. *Children Caring for Parents with Mental Illness: perspectives of young carers, parents and professionals.* Bristol: Policy Press; 2003.

8 Mueser KT, Fox L. A family intervention program for dual disorders. *Community Mental Health Journal.* 2002; **38**: 253–70.

9 Coulshed V. 'Engaging' in family therapy: problems for the inexperienced, uninvited therapist. *Journal of Family Therapy.* 1981; **3**: 51–8.

10 Prochaska JO, DiClemente CC, Norcross JC. In search of how people change: applications to addictive behaviors. *American Psychologist.* 1992; **47**: 1102–14.

11 Reupert A, Green K, Maybery D. Family care plans for families affected by parental mental illness. *Families in Society: The Journal of Contemporary Social Sciences.* 2008; **89**: 39–43.

12 Aguilera DC. *Crisis Intervention: theory and methodology.* 8th ed. St Louis, MO: Mosby; 1998.

13 Santisteban D. *Engaging Family Members into Adolescent Drug Treatment.* Florida Certification Board/Southern Coast Addiction Technology Transfer Center: Florida Department of Children and Families; 2009.

14 Stanhope V, Marcus S, Solomon P. The impact of coercion on services from the perspective of mental health care consumers with co-occurring disorders. *Psychiatric Services.* 2009; **60**: 183–8.

15 Westwood M, Pinzon J. Adolescent male health. *Paediatric Child Health.* 2008; **13**: 31–6.

16 O'Brien A, Fahmy R, Singh SP. Disengagement from mental health services: a literature review. *Social Psychiatry Psychiatric Epidemiology.* 2009; **44**: 558–68.

17 Padgett DK, Henwood B, Abrams C, *et al.* Engagement and retention in services among formerly homeless adults with co-occurring mental illness and substance abuse: voices from the margins. *Psychiatric Rehabilitation Journal.* 2008; **31**: 226–33.

18 Woolfall K, Sumnall H, McVeigh J. *Addressing the Needs of Children of Substance Using Parents: an evaluation of Families First's Intensive Intervention Final Report.* Liverpool: Centre for Public Health, John Moores University; 2008.

19 Wolfe BE, Goldfried MR. Research on psychotherapy integration: recommendations and conclusions from an NIMH workshop. *Journal of Consulting and Clinical Psychology.* 1988; **56**: 448–51.

20 Meier PS, Barrowclough C, Donmall MC. The role of the therapeutic alliance in the treatment of substance misuse: a critical review of the literature. *Addiction.* 2005; **100**: 304–16.

21 Trepka C, Rees A, Shapiro DA, *et al.* Therapist competence and outcome of cognitive therapy for depression. *Cognitive Therapy Research.* 2004; **28**: 143–57.

22 Young J. Online Distance Module 7: *Family Sensitive Practice in Mental Health Services.* Post Graduate Diploma of Community Psychiatric Nursing. Bendigo: Education Unit, La Trobe University; 1996. Available at: www.bouverie.org.au/research/bouverie-research-publications (accessed 30 September 2010).

23 Maybery D, Reupert A. Workforce capacity to respond to children whose parents have a mental illness. *Australian and New Zealand Journal of Psychiatry.* 2006; **40**: 657–64.

24 O'Grady CP, Skinner WJW. *Best Practices: concurrent mental health and substance use – partnering with families affected by concurrent disorders; facilitators' guide.* Vancouver: Health Canada; 2002.

25 Drake RE, Bartels SJ, Teague GB, *et al.* Treatment of substance abuse in severely mentally ill patients. *Journal of Nervous and Mental Disorders.* 1993; **181**: 606–11.

26 Diamond G, Josephson A. Family-based treatment research: a 10-year update. *Journal of the American Academy of Child and Adolescent Psychiatry.* 2005; **44**: 872–87.

27 Staiger P, Ricciardelli L, McCabe M. *Clients with a Dual Diagnosis: to what extent do they slip through the net?* Final report. Melbourne: Faculty of Health, Medicine, Nursing & Behavioural Sciences, Deakin University; 2008.

TO LEARN MORE

- Reupert A, Maybery D. *The Importance of Being Child and Family Focused.* 2007. Available at: www.copmi.net.au/gems/documents/copmigems01.pdf (accessed 23 January 2011).
- *Seven Principles of Family Sensitive Practice.* Available at: www.bouverie.org.au/programs/mental-health-team/family-sensitive-practive-family-sensitive-training/seven-principles (accessed 23 January 2011).
- Szirom T, King D, Desmond K. *Barriers to service provision for young people with presenting substance misuse and mental health problems.* National Youth Affairs Research Scheme; 2004. Accessed at: http://catalogue.nla.gov.au/Record/3424055 (accessed 23 January 2011).
- Woolfall K, Sumnall H, McVeigh J. *Addressing the Needs of Children of Substance Using Parents: an evaluation of Families First's Intensive Intervention;* 2008. Available at: www.cph.org.uk/showPublication.aspx?pubid=455 (accessed 23 January 2011).
- O'Grady CP, Skinner WJW. *Partnering with Families Affected by Concurrent Disorders: facilitators' guide.* Toronto: Centre for Addiction and Mental Health; 2007. Available at: www.camh.net/Publications/Resources_for_Professionals/Partnering_with_families/partnering_families_famguide.pdf (accessed 23 January 2011).
- O'Grady CP, Skinner WJW. *A Family Guide to Concurrent Disorders.* Toronto: Centre for Addiction and Mental Health; 2007. Available at: www.camh.net/Publications/Resources_for_Professionals/Partnering_with_families/partnering_families_facguide.pdf (accessed 23 January 2011).
- Dawe S, Harnett P, Frye S. *Improving Outcomes for Children Living in Families with Parental Substance Misuse: what do we know and what should we do.* Melbourne: Australian Institute of Family Studies; 2008. Available at: www.aifs.gov.au/nch/pubs/issues/issues29/issues29.pdf (accessed 23 January 2011).
- Scott D. Think child think family. *Family Matters Issue No. 81.* Australian Institute of Family Studies; 2009. Available at: www.aifs.gov.au/institute/pubs/fm2009/fm81/ds.pdf (accessed 23 January 2011).
- Children of Mentally Ill Consumers Family Support Kit. Available at: www.howstat.com/comic/Downloads/FamilyKit_2008.pdf (accessed 23 January 2011).
- **Families where a Parent has a Mental Illness (FaPMI)**
  The Department of Human Services' Mental Health Branch (Division of Mental Health and Drugs) developed a Service Development Strategy for Families where a Parent has a Mental Illness (FaPMI) in 2007. Available at: http://bouverie.org.au/programs/mental-health-team/fapmi and www.health.vic.gov.au/mentalhealth/families/index.htm (accessed 23 January 2011).

- **The Bouverie Centre**

  The Bouverie Centre, Victoria's Family focuses on the important role of the family and the power of relationships to foster social, emotional and mental well-being for at-risk individuals and their families and for the community. Available at: http://bouverie.org.au/ (accessed 23 January 2011).

- **Dual Diagnosis Australia and New Zealand**

  An online community of people interested in contributing to better outcomes for persons with co-occurring substance use and mental health disorders. On this site you will find dual diagnosis publications, training materials, capacity building and treatment resources and links to the most useful websites. Available at: www.dualdiagnosis.org.au/home/ (accessed 23 January 2011).

- **Children of Parents with a Mental Illness (COPMI) Resource Centre**

  This site has comprehensive information and resources for workers including teachers, parents, children and young people and families. This national project is based in Adelaide, Australia. Available at: www.copmi.net.au (accessed 23 January 2011).

- **Children who have a Parent with a Mental Illness (CHAMPS), aged 5–12**

  This website is for younger children to help them and their families understand mental illness. It has child-friendly information and links to resources for this age group. Available at: www.easternhealth.org.au/services/directory/service,serviceid,13789.aspx (accessed 23 January 2011).

- **Families and Dual Diagnosis**

  The New South Wales Department of Community Services has developed a comprehensive resource kit for working with children and families around issues of dual diagnosis. See website for ordering information. Available at: www.community.nsw.gov.au/about_us/news_and_publications/dual_diagnosis_resources.html (accessed 23 January 2011).

CHAPTER 8

Screening

Brian R Rush and Saulo Castel

INTRODUCTION

In this chapter, we focus on evidence-based screening for mental health–substance use disorders. We advocate for screening to be part of routine service delivery for adults as well as children and adolescents in a wide variety of service contexts, including, but not limited to, specialised mental health–substance use services. It is beyond the scope of this chapter to undertake a review of all the optional screening tools that have been developed. Such reviews are available for tools appropriate for adults[1,2] and children and adolescents.[3,4] We:

➤ review the rationale underlying recommendations for more proactive screening
➤ discuss the important distinction between screening and assessment and the need for a staged approach
➤ highlight different approaches to screening, several basic principles and constructs for evaluating the performance of screening tools, and practical aspects involved in application of these tools in practice settings
➤ offer some well-researched examples of tools for adolescents and adults that fit within the staged framework.

In closing, we discuss the need to shift from tool development and validation per se to the evaluation of screening tools in day-to-day practice and associated outcomes.

WHY MORE SYSTEMATIC SCREENING IS NEEDED

One of the strongest and most consistent recommendations across virtually all best practice syntheses and policy documents concerning mental health–substance use problems[5-7] has been the need for better screening processes to identify mental and/or substance use disorders among people presenting for help in a wide range of service settings. Best practice recommendations typically target managers and administrators of specialised mental health and substance use services and call for evidence-based screening for mental health disorders among people accessing substance use services and, vice versa, substance use screening among those accessing mental health services. However, better screening tools and processes for mental health and substance use are also needed in the wider health and social service delivery system – for example, various settings associated with the criminal justice system[8] as well as primary care and emergency services. To cite but one response to this identified need, prestigious organisations such as the American Medical Association[9] have recommended for some time that health professionals ask all adolescents about their use of alcohol and other drugs as part of their routine care. Similar recommendations have been made for screening and brief intervention with adults.

Much of the argument underlying the call for more systematic screening is based on the rationale for improved integration of services and systems for people experiencing mental health–substance use disorders. In this regard, screening is viewed as one component of a comprehensive approach to the design of better-integrated services and systems (*see* Book 3, Chapter 12). The rationale is based on research findings concerning the substantive overlap among people experiencing mental health–substance use disorders in the general population[10] – a large proportion of whom do not access mental health or substance use services[11,12] – and the fact that the overlap is associated with higher unmet need.[13] Studies in service delivery settings illustrate an even higher degree of overlap among these people compared with the general population,[14] and yet the vast majority of those experiencing mental health–substance use disorders are not identified[15,16] and are not receiving adequate treatment and support.[11,17] Better detection is seen as a first step towards a more integrated assessment and treatment response[18,19] and improved outcomes. Further, although the 'business case' for screening has not formally been developed in economic terms, there is an expectation that better detection, followed by integrated assessment and treatment and support, would reduce the high costs of serving people experiencing mental health–substance use disorders.[20] It should also reduce at least some of the barriers these people experience in navigating the historically disparate mental health and substance use systems.[21,22]

Beyond this general rationale for better detection and more integrated assessment and treatment, it has also been determined that not only are mental and substance use disorders often undetected through routine intake and assessment processes but also that well-validated screening tools are more effective than unstructured clinical interviews.[23,24]

KEY POINT 8.1

Screening tools are intended to complement rather than replace good clinical judgement.

A life-course perspective is also important in establishing the rationale for more routine and systematic screening of mental health–substance use disorders. That is to say, research on prevalence and impact of mental health–substance use disorders also considers the **trajectory** of mental and substance use problems and disorders over time (e.g. from childhood to adolescence and adolescence to young adulthood and beyond). Data from good-quality, population-based, longitudinal studies of children and adolescents are particularly relevant as they show many common risk factors for substance use and mental disorders, as well as the persistence of such disorders from adolescence to adulthood.[25]

The vast majority of substance use disorders in adolescence and young adulthood are predated by mental health problems in childhood or adolescence.[26-29]

These findings have considerable potential for prevention (e.g. bolstering the substance use component of parenting programmes for at-risk children), but depend on the successful detection of these problems at a young age.

All of the above constitute a strong rationale for more systematic screening for mental and/or substance use disorders. The case is quite strong with respect to adults. One might argue that the need is even more pressing among children and adolescents given the available evidence that early recognition and evidence-based treatment of substance use and mental health challenges could make a positive difference to the life course and future quality of life of those identified individuals. It follows that there is high interest in developing, and deploying in multiple service delivery sectors, validated screening tools that help professionals identify mental health–substance use disorders among children, adolescents and adults.

SCREENING VERSUS ASSESSMENT: A STAGED PROCESS

The terms 'screening' and 'assessment' can be confusing since the literature is not consistent in their use. There is a general consensus that screening and assessment are 'processes', both of which aim to measure and identify mental health and substance use-related needs, strengths and behaviours. However, some **screening** tools have the look and feel of more comprehensive assessment tools simply because they are lengthy and comprehensive in the coverage of disorders or problem domains (e.g. the Psychiatric Diagnostic Screening Questionnaire[30]). On the other hand, some **assessment** tools may actually be quite brief (and have the look and feel of a screening tool) if they focus only on a specific disorder (e.g. the Beck Depression Inventory[31]). Importantly, it is not the number of questions, or administration time, that make one tool a screener and another an assessment instrument; it depends on how it has been developed and validated, for what purpose, and how it is linked to further information gathering processes to confirm the findings.

It is also important to distinguish between the screening or assessment 'tool' and the screening or assessment 'process'. In service delivery settings, the application of a screening tool must fit seamlessly into the flow of individuals through intake procedures (sometimes by telephone); the routine scheduling of initial appointment(s) for assessment generally (sometimes on a drop-in basis but usually highly structured around one or two appointments of a specific duration); and other agency policies and practices for such things as whether the individual can be asked to take questionnaires home for completion between appointments. The questions must also be introduced in a way that is safe for the person to respond honestly, and enhances motivation to continue with the assessment and treatment and support planning process. Issues of literacy are also critically important as to whether the person needs support in completing self-administered screening tools.

A screening process is intended to be an efficient way of raising a 'red flag' about the possibility of a particular disorder or problem area, and thereby set the stage for a subsequent, more detailed assessment with a definite view to service planning and delivery. In a given service delivery setting, it would be a waste of scarce resources to implement a full-blown mental health and/or substance use assessment for all people presenting for assistance. Similarly, in a preventive context, it would be a waste of resources to implement preventive services for those who do not truly need them. In short, screening provides for 'economical identification' whereas assessment refers to more extensive and individualised identification of mental health and substance use strengths and needs of people whose screening results warrant future investigation.

It is helpful to conceptualise both screening and assessment as involving more than one step. For assessment, one step involves the process of gathering information for the purpose of understanding, and the next step, the actual diagnosis or problem definition for purposes of classification, and implementing evidence-based protocols specific to particular disorders or problem areas.[32] Assessment data also serve another important function as baseline information for the determination of outcome.[33] However, the most complex task in the assessment process is to investigate the interrelationship of the mental health disorders and the substance use disorders in terms of their interaction and aetiology. There are many ways in which alcohol and other drug use can interact with severe mental health problems; *see* references[33–36] for comprehensive discussions of the most salient issues, including Mueser and colleagues.[37] for a comprehensive discussion of aetiological theories.

There is cause for concern about the reliability of information from assessments conducted with people experiencing mental health–substance use disorders as with those with substance use disorders.[38] Some of these concerns are relevant to screening tools as well. There is evidence of lower reliability of self-reported past or current psychiatric disorders among people using drugs versus non-drug-using individuals.[39,40] There is also lower reliability of self-reported alcohol and drug use and consequences among people with severe mental illness, this being exacerbated by fluctuations in acute symptomatology, cognitive impairment and mental status.[35]

One of the strongest recommendations made by experts in the field is for assessment to be conducted over more than one interview, and to include multiple sources of information. In some ways this helps distinguish assessment from screening, although it may be advantageous in some circumstances to repeat screening tests on more than one occasion – for example, to help rule out disorders and problem areas significantly affected by heavy substance use. Thus, assessment must be seen as an **ongoing process** that extends over a period of time, including a period of abstinence or significant reduction in use.[33] This integrative, longitudinal approach is described by Drake and colleagues.[35] and Kranzler and colleagues.[41] the latter having formalised this integrative approach into the Longitudinal, Expert, All Data (LEAD) procedure. This integrates all information and observations about the individual that are available from multiple professionals, and over repeated assessments. Carey and Correia[33] note that this approach was found to be less effective for concurrent mood and anxiety disorders compared with other comorbidities. The longitudinal approach, however, is critical to sorting out the 'chicken-and-egg' problem. As noted by Carey and Correia,[33] if psychiatric symptoms continue during periods of abstinence this helps establish the diagnostic and statistical manual or mental disorders (DSM) criterion of 'not due to substance use'. Alternatively, the resolution of some or all of the psychiatric symptoms during periods of little or no use is consistent with a substance-induced disorder.

Returning to screening, it can also be conceptualised as involving two distinct steps. The first step is to identify the possibility of the person having **any** disorder (this objective is referred to as **case finding**), and this can be accomplished with one of several short instruments currently available (*see* DSM). The second step, however, involves screening tools that are typically longer and much more specific and that aim, in the one instrument, to tentatively identify one or more specific disorders (this objective is referred to as **case definition**). A stepped approach to

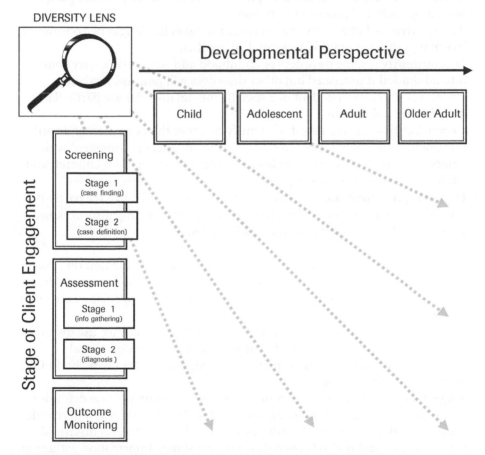

FIGURE 8.1 Framework for research, development and dissemination of screening tools for mental, substance use and mental health–substance use disorders

screening involves the sequential use of case-finding and case-definition tools, the objective being to reserve the more resource-intensive tools for those who score above the cut-off on a briefer, economical case-finding tool. When placed in the larger context of screening **and** assessment, such stage-one and stage-two screening tools would work together to ensure progressive but judicious and efficient use of assessment resources to guide treatment and support planning.

The top of the framework (Figure 8.1) highlights the need for screening tools to be developmentally appropriate. While it is usually taken as a given that screening tools designed for adults will not necessarily be appropriate for screening children and adolescents, less attention has been given to the special case of older adults (*see* Book 3, Chapter 5; Book 6, Chapter 11). Focusing on children and adolescents, Grisso and colleagues[8] point out that the developmental perspective seeks to describe and explain how the mental disorders of young people emerge and change over time (*see* Chapter 6; Book 3, Chapters 6 and 7; Book 6, Chapters 12 and 13). Thus, mental disorders of adolescents, including substance use disorders, are not just 'older' versions of childhood disorders; neither are they 'less mature' versions of adult disorders. They cite the main implications of the developmental perspective for screening tools and processes as being:

➤ **Age relativity** – behaviours, emotions or thoughts that might be considered 'normal' at one age may be 'abnormal' at another.
➤ **Discontinuity** – some disorders of childhood and adolescence may continue into adulthood if untreated but other disorders will not, and further, emotional states independent of a specific mental disorder are particularly unstable in adolescence.
➤ **Comorbidity** – the likelihood of identifying more than one mental disorder is thought to be much higher in children and adolescents compared with adults; this may be a function of how disorders are defined for children and adolescents, and/or that their psychopathology is just more complex.
➤ **Demographic differences** – factors such as gender difference are particularly critical (e.g. boys are more likely to experience externalising disorders and girls more likely to experience internalising disorders).

The left side of the framework highlights the staged approach based on phases of engagement, an aspect of the framework specific to screening for mental health–substance use disorders with people in contact with helping agencies. Screening is seen in two stages:

➤ **Stage One** is focused on case finding for mental and substance use disorders but, importantly, also screening for other health problems of critical importance to treatment and support planning, such as traumatic brain injury or cognitive impairment.
➤ **Stage Two** is focused on more comprehensive screening for case definition – that is, specific substance use and/or mental disorders such as a psychotic disorder, major depressive disorder or cocaine dependence. As discussed earlier, assessment is also broken down to two stages: information gathering and diagnosis/classification for purposes of treatment and support planning. The last stage is one of outcome monitoring, an area that is currently

underdeveloped in the mental health and substance use field, insofar as the links to screening and assessment from both measurement and practical viewpoints need to be better defined. Recent developments in the substance use area that consider outcome monitoring as a continuous process that occurs during treatment as well as after treatment[42] is a major step forward in conceptualising and operationalising the links among screening, assessment and outcome monitoring.

The last aspect of the framework is the 'diversity lens' through which one must consider both the developmental trajectory and the process of engagement. This calls attention to the special cultural and other diversity-related perspectives that need to be brought to bear when conducting research on screening and assessment tools and processes, and also when implementing and interpreting various tools in the context of day-to-day practice (*see* Chapter 5; Book 1, Chapter 5; Book 4, Chapters 4 and 5).

DIFFERENT APPROACHES TO SCREENING

Mental health disorders or problems, including substance use disorders/problems, may present in a less differentiated, less specific way with children and adolescents than with adults and older people. Thus, there are different approaches by which those disorders and problems are identified and classified, and this has major implications for how screening (and assessment) tools are constructed. These approaches, which can also be used for adults, include:

➤ A categorical, **diagnostic approach** based on DSM (DSM-IV-TR).[43] This is the predominant system currently in place within our health system and is closely linked to evidence-based practices for clinical interventions, as well as to the design of new research to improve clinical practice on an ongoing basis.

➤ A **dimensional approach** in which individuals are assessed along different dimensions, which can enrich the information conveyed by the categorical approach. Examples of currently used dimensions are:

 — A **symptom-based** approach, whereby children and adolescents are screened on the basis of symptoms but not necessarily in the context of specific diagnoses. Examples would include anger, depressed mood, frequent alcohol or drug use, or worry.

 — A **behavioural** approach that seeks to describe behaviours that may or may not align with specific psychiatric diagnostic categories. Perhaps the best-known model was developed by Achenbach – namely, the two broad groupings of internalising and externalising disorders. The GAIN-Short Screener (GSS) is a recent example of a dimensional screening tool including internalising and externalising disorders.[44]

 — The **problem-oriented** approach, which targets strengths and weaknesses in functioning of day-to-day living such as family and peer relations, school, social activities and/or alcohol or drug use and related difficulties. Some tools using a problem-oriented approach for children and adolescents also frame it as risk assessment.

Since the categorical diagnostic approach is so firmly embedded in current clinical guidelines and ongoing research, the dimensional approaches should be seen as complementary to a categorical approach and not as replacements.

BASIC PRINCIPLES AND PROCEDURES FOR EVALUATING SCREENING PROCEDURES OR TESTS

When evaluating screening tools, two of the psychometric properties of those procedures – reliability and validity – are usually taken into account. Within this context, reliability can be defined as the consistency of the result ('caseness' or not) as obtained by different raters (interrater reliability) or at different times (test–retest reliability), and using the same instrument.[45] Reliability is a *sine-qua-non* condition for the usefulness of any screening procedure, which is to say that an unreliable procedure is useless and there is no point in engaging in further discussions of its applicability.

There are many types of validity and for the purposes of this chapter a specific type, criterion validity, is the most relevant. It can be defined as the extent to which a screening instrument renders the same diagnosis (or caseness) obtained by a 'gold standard', the latter usually being a structured or semi-structured diagnostic interview administered by a trained interviewer, or sometimes the judgement of an experienced professional informed by the best available information about a potential case. The controversy about the 'gold standard' in mental health and substance use test development is beyond the scope of this chapter. Validity has been referred to as a property of the screening test but is better conceptualised as a property of a procedure, as it pertains to the use of a screening test in a given context, for a specific purpose.[46] Thus, on screening for mental health or substance use disorders among any given population, the question becomes: 'Is this screening test valid among individuals belonging to this specific population?' – as opposed to the more generic question: 'Is this screening test valid?'[47]

Predictive validity, which refers to the assessment of future status of a particular construct based on current status, as measured by the screening tool, can be understood as a particular case of criterion validity in which the criterion will take place in the future. An example would be predicting alcohol or drug dependence as a young adult, based on results obtained from a screening tool administered at age ten.

Much research on validation of screening tools, including that of the authors, is based on constructs closely related to diagnostic criteria and formal DSM-based diagnoses because of their predominant and critical role in current clinical guidelines, treatment planning and ongoing research. In other words, the focus in the screening literature has been on criterion-related validity with DSM diagnoses as the gold standard. This has the advantage of allowing one to compare performance of different screening tools, since one has a common and widely accepted gold standard, at least for adults. Several experts in child and adolescent psychiatry acknowledge the limitations of current DSM-based diagnoses for children and adolescents.

For readers interested in a more detailed discussion about the psychometric properties of screening tools, we recommend Grisso and colleagues[8] and Streiner and Norman.[48]

PRACTICAL ASPECTS OF SCREENING AND ASSESSMENT PROCESSES

Not only do effective screening and assessment tools need to be guided by good psychometric test development and evaluation but also the expectation and over-all performance of a given test is highly dependent on the context in which it is implemented. From a systems point of view there are many doorways into mental health and/or substance use services and supports. While this obviously includes specialised services, it also includes more generic services and community organi-sations such as:

➤ primary care, including emergency services
➤ family and children's services
➤ social assistance
➤ justice-related programmes and institutions
➤ schools.

For people presenting to specialised substance use services it is probably safe to say that a screening tool for substance use disorders is not needed. There is, however, a great need for a screening tool to help identify mental disorders given the likelihood of mental health problems that have not been identified. Similarly, a screening tool for substance use disorders is probably needed with people presenting to mental health services. Further, there is value in using the same screening tool in both types of services insofar as that tool is able to perform both functions (referred to as a 'dual-function' screening tool). This gives local mental health and substance use professionals a common language and common set of information through which to facilitate development of better-integrated services. Also, in these specialised mental health and substance use services, there may be considerably more enthusi-asm for screening because of the high priority attached to mental health–substance use disorders in recent years, and the well-known impact of these disorders on retention and treatment outcome. Specifically, these specialised settings may be more motivated to implement the staged screening and assessment process identi-fied earlier, and commit to the longer, more comprehensive screening tools than might be practicable for more generic health and social services.

Once a person becomes engaged with a particular service or service delivery system there will be different pathways and 'checkpoints' through the intake, assessment, treatment and support planning process that present as opportunities for screening. A common checkpoint is the intake interview; another is the begin-ning of the assessment phase itself. Screening, or repeat screening, may also be something that is held off until the person has sufficiently stabilised so as to ensure meaningful results (e.g. following crisis intervention or detoxification services). This would depend on the severity and urgency of the overall presenting situation.

The nature of the target population seen in various service delivery settings and, in particular, the age range of the population, will be critical to the selection of the screening tools. The younger the age of the person the greater the need to use tools that require completion by a parent or perhaps a teacher.

Grisso and colleagues[8] emphasise that a service considering the implementation of a screening process for mental and/or substance use disorders should clearly

articulate the purpose(s) to which the results will be put. They identify three main objectives:
1 improving professional decision-making
2 fulfilling regulatory requirements and professional standards
3 managing resources.

Improving professional decision-making

Expectation of improved professional decisions is the most common motivator for implementing a standard screening process, and typically with short-term management strategies in mind for the person requiring services or supports. This goal relates back to the value of a multistage screening and assessment process as an aid to individualised, treatment and support planning. Indirectly, this also speaks to the need for training in the use of the tool, as well as the need for good manuals and instructions for administration. If the goal in choosing a screening tool is to minimise the need for special qualifications or training to use the tool, this will depend on how structured it is (i.e. how fixed or flexible the format for test administration), as well as the simplicity of the tool itself (i.e. response categories and scoring procedures). Typically, 'cut-off' scores for a given tool become part of the clinical decision-making process, but tools vary widely with respect to compu-terised versus manual scoring and the extent to which results may be 'normed' for different subgroups – for example, males versus females.

KEY POINT 8.3

It is essential that the plan for using the results of a screening tool is prepared and documented in policy and procedures. Moreover, the latter need to be widely communicated and adequately monitored and reinforced.

Regulatory requirements and professional standards

Different types of services may have regulatory requirements to screen for spe-cific types of problems (e.g. suicide risk or other safety needs). If the service has a lengthy list of other health and social conditions that must be screened for, there will likely be more pressure to keep the screening tool for mental and/or substance use disorders brief.

Managing resources

Managing resources is the third mentioned area. Examples would include adjusting professional complements and skills to ensure coverage in particular topic areas, ensuring adequate linkages are in place with outside agencies for certain types of problems areas, and lobbying for additional funding.

Other factors

In addition to these factors, there is the link to outcome monitoring as highlighted in the framework presented here. Some, but not all, screening tools can serve this function. If the items are properly structured (e.g. aimed at symptoms or concerns that are changeable), and if the content is linked to the actual services that have been provided, it should be possible to link the screening function with outcome assessment. If not, this link to future outcome monitoring is something that should be done within the assessment stage.

Another, less frequently discussed aspect of the clinical application of a screening tool is the relationship between the use of a screening tool and the process of engagement, motivation and therapeutic alliance. An effective screening process depends on having a good tool to use, but also on the competence of the professional to use it with individuals in a non-threatening and engaging manner.

These various reasons for implementing a systematic and universal screening do not all need to be addressed in a given application of a screening tool. One or more may be the primary reasons and the other factors may be less important, or perhaps not viewed as important at all.

Contextual factors associated with implementing a screening tool include the **organisational context** as this can govern access to tools that are available through copyright only – for example, those available only on a pay-per-use basis. Other contextual factors relate to whether adequate computer and information technology exists to support computerised administration of particular tools and to access automated scoring and feedback via the Internet. As noted earlier, the computer is playing a much bigger role in screening processes and is the subject of considerable research.[49] Finally, the level of expertise required for administration, scoring and interpretation of some tools will vary significantly across service delivery settings. Stage Two screening tools for case definition will require more training and expertise than the briefer tools for case finding (Stage One).

Lastly, there are factors related to policy and research. Policy-related factors may lie within the organisation (e.g. adjusting internal policies related to the flow of individuals through the internal delivery pathway),[50] or with service delivery partners (e.g. calling for interagency agreements on how people with particular problems or disorders will be case-managed or referred – *see* Book 2, Chapters 8, 9, 11 and 12). Internal policy issues also determine the extent to which it is mandatory for all professionals to use the screening tool(s) on a routine basis. It is the experience of the authors that some will be 'pro-tool' while others strongly oppose their use, typically on the grounds that tools interfere with establishing good rapport with individuals and their families. Although the factors underlying these differences in perception are not well understood, the differences are critically important for systematic and sustainable use of virtually any tool regardless of its psychometric performance. Policy also comes into play at a regional, provincial/state or even national level; for example, when a policy mandates that funded programmes will use a particular screening tool for purposes of consistency in communication, public health surveillance and perhaps performance monitoring. Research objectives may also be in play, such as monitoring trends over time in the characteristics of service recipients compared with the general population. Policy issues also abound with respect to not only the use of the results but also whether, and how, others can access the results for purposes other than what was intended.

SELECTED SCREENING TOOLS FOR MENTAL AND SUBSTANCE USE DISORDERS

In this section, we highlight three screening tools that fit within the staged model of screening and assessment. All three are 'dual-function' tools, that is, they screen for substance use disorders/problems as well as other mental health disorders/problems. The first, the GAIN-SS[44] is a Stage One screener appropriate for ages 12 and over. The second, the DISC Predictive Scales (DPS)[51] is a Stage Two screener appropriate for children and adolescents between the ages of 9 and 17. The third, the Psychiatric Diagnostic Screening Questionnaire (PDSQ),[24,30] is a Stage Two screener appropriate for transitional youth and adults 18 years of age and over. Thus, with these three tools, one can implement the two-staged screening model from ages 12 and up with confidence in the validation data behind the tools.

GAIN-Short Screener (GAIN-SS)

The first tool we highlight is the GAIN-SS.[44] This instrument is a brief, 3- to 5-minute screening tool comprising 20 items divided into four five-item subscales. The tool is part of a family of screening and assessment measures related to the Global Appraisal of Individual Needs (GAIN – www.chestnut.org). Four subscales are identified for internalising disorders, externalising disorders, substance use disorders and crime/violence (*see* Book 3, Chapter 14; Book 6, Chapter 14). This relatively new screener has attracted considerable attention among policymakers and programme managers, in part because of its brevity, its coverage of the two broad domains of psychopathology (internalising and externalising disorders), as well as substance use. Thus, it is a dual-function tool that has high potential as a common tool for substance use services (to screen for mental disorders) and for mental health services (to screen for substance use disorders). Its brevity and coverage also make it a good option for primary care and other generic health and social services. GAIN-SS responses are given in terms of the recency of the problem described in the questions: 3 = past month; 2 = 2–12 months ago; 1 = 1+ years ago; 0 = never. The number of past-month symptoms (number of 3s) is used as a measure of change; the number of past-year symptoms (number of 3s and 2s) is used to identify who is likely to have a current diagnosis; and the number of lifetime symptoms (total of 3s, 2s and 1s) is used as a covariate measure of lifetime severity.

The original validation data for the GAIN-SS are derived from a study that pools information for over 6000 adolescents and almost 2000 adults from multiple locations across the United States. The initial validation work involved an assessment of the congruence of the GAIN-SS in determining the diagnostic results (i.e. impressions) derived from the full GAIN bio-psychosocial assessment. This design yielded excellent specificity and sensitivity for both adults and adolescents but further work was called for in validating the results of the GAIN-SS with independent diagnostic criteria. This work has recently been conducted by the authors and the performance of the instrument was satisfactory and comparable with the other brief, case-finding screening tools that were also assessed.[52] The tool is available at low cost through Chestnut Health Systems – www.chestnut.org (accessed 23 January 2011).

Psychiatric Diagnostic Screening Questionnaire

The PDSQ is a comprehensive 111-item screening tool for specific Axis I disorders designed for self-administration, with no supplementary clinical interview component.[23,30] The 111 items are comprised of 13 sets of yes/no questions, each set corresponding to a diagnostic category aligned with DSM-IV. The number of items in each set of questions varies, with a high of 21 items in the depressive module and a low of five items in the hypochondriasis section. The time period for reporting varies by item set, with some sets, such as the depressive module, based on the past two weeks, and others, such as psychosis, based on the past six months. Scoring occurs within each set of items (1 = yes, 0 = no) and these are summed for each subscale. Completion time is approximately 15–20 minutes. The PDSQ covers the most prevalent Axis I mental disorders in DSM-IV and has undergone extensive test development procedures including readability, understandability, reliability and validity testing.[24,30] The accuracy in predicting subsequent psychiatric diagnoses has been replicated among substance-using individuals drawn from a psychiatric outpatient population.[53] The authors have recently found a satisfactory level of test performance directly in a heterogeneous sample of people seeking specialised treatment for substance use.[52] The copyright on the PDSQ is held by Western Psychological Services and the tool is available on a pay-per-use basis (email: customerservice@wpspublish.com).

DISC Predictive Scales

The DPS is an instrument comprised of a diagnosis-specific self-report inventory designed to identify youth endorsing symptoms and who are highly likely to meet diagnostic criteria. The scales and related items are derived from a secondary analysis of a large epidemiological dataset containing responses to the full Diagnostic Interview Schedule for Children (DISC-2.3) and other DSM-III diagnostic information. The total number of items is 56 and they refer to the past 12 months. Subscales include simple phobia, social phobia, agoraphobia, overanxious disorder, obsessive–compulsive disorder, separation anxiety disorder, eating disorders, major depressive disorder, attention deficit hyperactivity disorder (ADHD), oppositional defiant disorder, conduct disorder and alcohol/substance use disorder. There is a youth version and a parent version.

Although the tool is comparatively new, we located three studies that validated the tool against a diagnostic gold standard.[51,54,55] Two were based in a youth correctional facility and one from a community high school sample. The validation methods and results were good to excellent in predicting specific disorders, including substance use disorders. Results were a bit more modest in the community sample (which one might expect), but still quite good. McReynolds and colleagues[54] reported excellent results with respect to internal consistency. Administration options include parent and youth self-report and the instrument is typically delivered via computer with items appearing on the screen and also heard by audio via headphones. A PDF copy of the tool is available at no cost from the author (C Lucas) and the software version is available by email (casiasoftware@optonline.net) at a cost set at that time.

SUMMARY AND CONCLUSION

The call for the routine and widespread use of screening tools for mental health–substance use disorders is a core element of the movement towards more integrated mental health and substance use services and systems. The rationale is strong for more effective screening tools to be developed and applied across the age span and multiple service delivery sectors. Much is known about the methods of test development and validation, and there is no shortage of well-validated tools, many of which fit well with a staged model of screening and assessment. Linking screening tools to subsequent outcome monitoring is an area that needs more research and development, as is the need for more work with tools for older populations and tools that are culturally sensitive. That said, given the availability of so many excellent and well-validated tools, the work in this important area needs to shift somewhat to the evaluation of using screening tools in various practice settings and the outcomes associated with this. Such outcomes are likely to be evident at the person, programme and community-systems levels. This is a topic area ripe for drawing upon the emerging field of implementation science.

ACKNOWLEDGEMENTS

The authors would like to thank many of our colleagues at the Centre for Addiction and Mental Health who have worked with us on the validation and dissemination of a range of screening tools for mental health and substance use disorders and the review and synthesis of research information on screening tools applicable to children and adolescents. We would like to thank Renée Desmond in particular for her excellent support on many of these projects and, most recently, in the preparation of this chapter specifically.

REFERENCES

1 Sacks S. Brief overview of screening and assessment for co-occurring disorders. *International Journal of Mental Health and Addiction.* 2008; **6**: 7–19.

2 Rush BR. On the screening and assessment of mental disorders among clients seeking help from specialized substance abuse treatment services: an international symposium. [Editorial]. *International Journal of Mental Health and Addiction.* 2008; **6**: 1–6.

3 Winters KC, Stinchfield R, Bukstein OG. Assessing adolescent substance use and abuse. In: Kaminer Y, Bukstein OG, editors. *Adolescent Substance Abuse: psychiatric comorbidity and high-risk behaviors.* New York: Routledge; 2008. pp. 53–86.

4 Rush BR, Castel S, Somers J, *et al.* Systematic review and research synthesis of screening tools for mental and substance use disorders appropriate for children and adolescents: technical report. Unpublished manuscript; May 2009.

5 Substance Abuse and Mental Health Services Administration. *Report to Congress on the Prevention and Treatment of Co-occurring Substance Abuse Disorders and Mental Disorders.* Washington, DC: Department of Health and Human Services; 2002.

6 Health Canada. Best *Practices: concurrent mental health and substance use disorders.* Ottawa, ON: Health Canada; 2001.

7 Baldacchino A, Corkery J. *Comorbidity: perspectives across Europe.* London: European Collaborative Centres in Addiction Studies; 2006.

8 Grisso T, Vincent G, Seagrave D. *Mental Health Screening and Assessment in Juvenile Justice.* New York: Guilford Press; 2005.

9 Elster AB, Kuznets NJ, editors. *American Medical Association Guidelines for Adolescent Preventive Services (GAPS).* Baltimore, MD: Williams & Wilkins; 1994.

10 Jané-Llopis E, Matytsina I. Mental health and alcohol, drugs and tobacco: a review of the comorbidity between mental disorders and the use of alcohol, tobacco and illicit drugs. *Drug and Alcohol Review.* 2006; **25**: 515–36.

11 Watkins KE, Burnam A, Kung F, et al. A national survey of care for persons with co-occurring mental and substance use disorders. *Psychiatric Services.* 2001; **52**: 1062–8.

12 Harris KM, Edlund MJ. Use of mental health care and substance abuse treatment among adults with co-occurring disorders. *Psychiatric Services.* 2005; **56**: 954–9.

13 Urbanoski KA, Rush BR, Wild TC, et al. Use of mental health care services by Canadians with co-occurring substance dependence and mental disorders. *Psychiatric Services.* 2007; **58**: 962–9.

14 Chan YF, Dennis ML, Funk RR. Prevalence and comorbidity of major internalizing and externalizing disorders among adolescents and adults presenting to substance abuse treatment. *Journal of Substance Abuse Treatment.* 2008; **34**: 14–24.

15 Ananth J, Vandewater S, Kamal M, et al. Missed diagnosis of substance abuse in psychiatric patients. *Hospital and Community Psychiatry.* 1989; **40**: 297–9.

16 Barnaby B, Drummond C, McCloud A, et al. Substance misuse in psychiatric inpatients: comparison of a screening questionnaire survey with case notes. *British Medical Journal.* 2003; **327**: 783–4.

17 Rush BR, Koegl CJ. Prevalence and profile of people with co-occurring mental and substance use disorders within a comprehensive mental health system. *Canadian Journal of Psychiatry.* 2008; **53**: 810–21.

18 Drake RE, O'Neal EL, Wallach MA. A systematic review of psychosocial research on psychosocial interventions for people with co-occurring severe mental and substance use disorders. *Journal of Substance Abuse Treatment.* 2008; **34**: 123–38.

19 Rush B, Fogg B, Nadeau L, et al. *On the Integration of Mental Health and Substance Use Services and Systems.* Ottawa, ON: Canadian Executive Council on Addictions; 2008.

20 Bartels SJ, Teague GB, Drake RE, et al. Substance abuse in schizophrenia: service utilization and costs. *Journal of Nervous and Mental Disease.* 1993; **181**: 227–32.

21 Ridgely MS, Goldman HH, Willenbring M. Barriers to the care of persons with dual diagnosis: organizational and financing issues. *Schizophrenia Bulletin.* 1990; **16**: 123–32.

22 Kay-Lambkin FJ, Baker AL, Lewin TJ. The 'co-morbidity roundabout': a framework to guide assessment and intervention strategies and engineer change among people with co-morbid problems. *Drug and Alcohol Review.* 2004; **23**: 407–23.

23 Zimmerman M. What should the standard of care for psychiatric diagnostic evaluations be? *Journal of Nervous and Mental Disease.* 2003; **191**: 281–6.

24 Zimmerman M, Mattia JI. A self-report to help make psychiatric diagnosis. the psychiatric diagnostic screening questionnaire. *Archives of General Psychiatry.* 2001; **58**: 787–94.

25 Adair CE. *Concurrent Substance Use and Mental Disorders in Adolescents: a review of the literature on current science and practice.* Calgary: Alberta Centre for Child Family and Community Research; 2009.

26 Merikangas KR, Avenevoli S. Implications of genetic epidemiology for the prevention of substance use disorders. *Addictive Behaviors.* 2000; **25**: 807–20.

27 Wise BK, Cuffe SP, Fischer T. Dual diagnosis and successful participation of adolescents in substance abuse treatment. *Journal of Substance Abuse Treatment.* 2001; **21**: 161–5.

28 Costello EJ, Mustillo S, Erkanli A, *et al*. Prevalence and development of psychiatric disorders in childhood and adolescence. *Archives of General Psychiatry*. 2003; **60**: 837–44.

29 Compton SN, Burns BJ, Egger HL, *et al*. Review of the evidence base for treatment of childhood psychopathology: internalizing disorders. *Journal of Consulting and Clinical Psychology*. 2002; **70**: 1240–66.

30 Zimmerman M, Mattia JI. The psychiatric diagnostic screening questionnaire: development, reliability and validity. *Comprehensive Psychiatry*. 2001; **42**: 175–89.

31 Beck AT, Ward CH, Mendelson M, *et al*. An inventory for measuring depression. *Archives of General Psychiatry*. 1961; **4**: 561–71.

32 Keaney F. Assessment and screening. *Psychiatry*. 2006; **5**: 431–6.

33 Carey KB, Correia CJ. Severe mental illness and addictions: assessment considerations. *Addictive Behaviors*. 1998; **23**: 735–48.

34 Ries R. *Assessment and Treatment of Patients with Coexisting Mental Illness and Alcohol and Other Drug Abuse: treatment improvement protocol (TIP) series 9*. DHHS Publication No. (SMA) 94–2078). Rockville, MD: Centre for Substance Abuse Treatment; 1994.

35 Drake RE, Osher FC, Noordsy DL, *et al*. Diagnosis of alcohol use disorders in schizophrenia. *Schizophrenia Bulletin*. 1990; **16**: 57–67.

36 Teitelbaum LM, Carey KB. Alcohol assessment in psychiatric patients. *Clinical Psychology: Science and Practice*. 1996; **3**: 323–38.

37 Mueser KT, Drake RE, Wallach MA. Dual diagnosis: a review of etiological theories. *Addictive Behaviors*. 1998; **23**: 717–34.

38 Del Boca F, Noll JA. Truth or consequences: the validity of self-report data in health services research on addictions. *Addiction*. 2000; **95**: S347–S360.

39 Bryant KL, Rounsaville B, Spitzer RL, *et al*. Reliability of dual diagnosis: substance dependence and psychiatric disorders. *Journal of Nervous and Mental Disorders*. 1992; **180**: 251–7.

40 Corty E, Lehman AF, Meyers CP. Influence of psychoactive substance use on the reliability of psychiatric diagnosis. *Journal of Consulting and Clinical Psychology*. 1993; **61**: 165–70.

41 Kranzler HR, Kadden RM, Babor TF, *et al*. Longitudinal, Expert, All Data procedure for psychiatric diagnosis in patients with psychoactive substance use disorders. *Journal of Nervous and Mental Disorders*. 1994; **182**: 277–83.

42 McLellan AT, McKay JR, Forman R, *et al*. Reconsidering the evaluation of addiction treatment: from retrospective follow-up to concurrent recovery monitoring. *Addiction*. 2005; **100**: 447–58.

43 American Psychiatric Association. *Diagnostic and Statistical Manual of Mental Disorders*. 4th ed. Text Revision. Washington, DC: American Psychiatric Association; 2000.

44 Dennis ML, Chan YF, Funk RR. Development and validation of the GAIN Short Screener (GSS) for internalizing, externalizing and substance use disorders and crime/violence problems among adolescents and adults. *American Journal on Addictions*. 2006; **15**: 80–91.

45 Blacker D, Endicott J. Psychometric properties: concepts of reliability and validity. In: Rush AJ Jr, First MB, Blacker D, editors. *Handbook of Psychiatric Measures*. Washington: American Psychiatric Association; 2000. pp. 7–14.

46 Streiner DL, Norman GR. 'Precision' and 'accuracy': two terms that are neither. *Journal of Clinical Epidemiology*. 2006; **59**: 327–30.

47 Castel S, Rush BR, Scalco MZ. Screening of mental disorders among clients with addictions: the need for population-specific validation. *International Journal of Mental Health and Addiction*. 2008; **6**: 64–71.

48 Streiner DL, Norman GR. *Health Measurement Scales: a practical guide to their development and use*. 4th ed. Oxford: Oxford University Press; 2008.

49 Knight JR, Harris SK, Sherritt L, *et al.* Adolescents' preferences for substance abuse screening in primary care practice. *Substance Abuse.* 2007; **28**: 107–17.

50 Sibley L. Integrating screening and assessment tools into clinical practice: where the rubber hits the road. *International Journal of Mental Health and Addiction.* 2008; **6**: 131–6.

51 Lucas CP, Zhang H, Fisher PW, *et al.* The DISC predictive scales (DPS): efficiently screening for diagnoses. *Journal of the American Academy of Child & Adolescent Psychiatry.* 2001; **40**: 443–9.

52 Rush BR, Castel S, Brands B, *et al. Validation and Comparison of Screening Tools for Mental Disorders in Substance Abusers.* San Juan, Puerto Rico: Presented to the 2008 annual meeting of the College on Problems of Drug Dependence; 2008.

53 Zimmerman M, Sheeran T, Chelminski I, *et al.* Screening for psychiatric disorders in outpatients with DSM-IV substance use disorders. *Journal of Substance Abuse Treatment.* 2004; **26**: 181–8.

54 McReynolds LS, Wasserman GA, Fisher P, *et al.* Diagnostic screening with incarcerated youths: comparing the DPS and Voice DISC. *Criminal Justice and Behavior.* 2007; **34**: 830–45.

55 Roberts N, Stuart H, Lam M. High school mental health survey: assessment of a mental health screen. *Canadian Journal of Psychiatry.* 2008; **53**: 314–22.

TO LEARN MORE

- Rush BR. On the screening and assessment of mental disorders among clients seeking help from specialized substance abuse treatment services: an international symposium. [Editorial]. *International Journal of Mental Health and Addiction.* 2008; **6**: 1–6. (This editorial introduces an issue of this journal that is devoted to the topic of screening and assessment of concurrent disorders).

- Chestnut Health Systems. Available at: www.chestnut.org. This website provides links to the family of screening and assessment instruments related to the GAIN-SS.

- Ries R. (Consensus panel chair). *Assessment and Treatment of Patients with Coexisting Mental Illness and Alcohol and Other Drug Abuse.* Treatment Improvement Protocol (TIP) Series No. Rockville, MD: Centre for Substance Abuse Treatment. DHHS Publication No. (SMA) 94–2078; 1994. Available at: www.health.org/pubs/catalog/ordering.htm (accessed 23 January 2011).

- Carey KB, Correia CJ. Severe mental illness and addictions: assessment considerations. *Addictive Behaviors.* 1998; **23**: 735–48.

CHAPTER 9

Assessment

Michael Adams and Gemma Stacey-Emile

PRE-READING EXERCISE 9.1

Time: 10 minutes

Consider in what ways an assessment process can be helpful to:

- you
- other intra- and interdisciplinary team members
- the individual and family.

Case study 9.1: Tom

Tom (22) lives with his parents. As a youth, Tom was a talented sportsman. He excelled at a variety of sports and activities, and was actively supported by his parents. Tom's academic progress was unremarkable but he obtained a college place to study for a sports diploma. From the age of 17 his behaviour began to change. He became disinterested in training and his studies deteriorated. He eventually stopped sports participation altogether and dropped out of college. His long-term girlfriend finished their relationship and he has not had a partner since.

Tom was already a social drinker and had been smoking cannabis for about two years. Gradually his consumption of these substances increased. He drifted away from his sporting friends, found a new peer group and became influenced by their behaviour. Tom and family give little account of what happened over the next couple of years other than an impression that he became gradually less sociable and more socially isolated. His mother became used to buying him beer and videos, and on one occasion paid off a debt when a drug dealer threatened him. Tom has by now developed a large tolerance for alcohol.

Tom starts to express ideation that someone is out to 'get' him and his family. He believes that he is being spied upon. The general practitioner arranges for him to be assessed at the local psychiatric unit and he is admitted, only to abscond and return home within hours. His parents decide not to encourage him to return to hospital. However, on the advice of the psychiatrist, his general practitioner prescribes a small dose of antipsychotic medication. Tom is reluctant to comply with this because it makes him feel drowsy, even though he continues to have paranoid ideation. His parents are extremely anxious about the situation, his mother follows him around the house 'in case he does something stupid', and both parents say repeatedly that 'something needs to be done'!

INTRODUCTION

There is a growing body of evidence indicating that there are numerous people like Tom in the United Kingdom (UK) presenting with mental health–substance use problems.[1,2] Estimates of the incidence vary, beginning at approximately one-third[1] but rising significantly among specific populations such as young men[1] and individuals with a forensic history.[3] It is generally accepted that people with mental health–substance use issues have additional difficulties to people with mental health problems who do not use substances; but due to a variety of complex physical, psychological, social and cultural issues it is often difficult to ascertain the precise nature of the relationship between mental health problems and substance use. However, it is generally accepted that increased rates of substance use will be found among persons with mental health problems, and higher rates of mental health problems will be found among persons who use substances.[4] Analysis of the available evidence has led the UK government to associate the problem with a variety of deleterious outcomes including:

➤ worsening psychiatric symptoms
➤ increased use of institutional services
➤ poor medication adherence
➤ homelessness
➤ increased risk of HIV infection
➤ poor social outcomes including impact on carers and family
➤ contact with the criminal justice system.[5]

While specific guidance has been issued regarding the management of illicit substances in UK inpatient settings,[6] there is a paucity of similar advice available to community professionals. Perhaps it is easier to construct guidance that involves reducing the consumption and free movement of substances within managed premises than in people's own homes where professionals are guests, and their ability to control what goes on is reduced considerably. In the case study, Tom's mother buys him alcohol to consume in the home in the belief that this is better than him venturing out to purchase substances. Various explanations have been offered as to why people with mental health–substance use problems are difficult to engage in community settings including:

➤ poor communication among services
➤ unrealistic contracts and boundaries
➤ disruptive relationships
➤ risk management issues
➤ avoidant workers and services

➤ moralistic views
➤ lack of cohesive team working.[7]

However, some commentators have cautioned against the proliferation of research that concentrates on the negative connotations associated with the problem, which they believe may contribute to a lowering of optimism in treatment.[8] Yet recent literature does not entirely paint such a pessimistic picture; it has been shown that commitment to structural integrity of services, targeted training of certain professional groups and ongoing supervision can give cause for optimism.[9]

It has been known for some time that in a UK context and particularly in the region where the authors practise (Wales), the most prominent problem is that of concurrent mental health problems and alcohol use.[1] The assessment and engagement issues presented by Tom in the case study could be viewed as typical of the types of challenges presented to professionals. Therefore, the remainder of this chapter examines the assessment considerations that come into play in the engagement of people with mental health problems and excessive alcohol use within a predominately community setting, and provides a context for discussion.

CONTEXTUAL BACKGROUND

In its simplest form, the care of individuals with mental health–substance use problems brings together different professional activities which may have contradictory treatment philosophies. Yet even within these separate fields of practice different values and beliefs abound, and this, in conjunction with the individual's own unique circumstances, introduces a complexity that rejects notions that care can be delivered in a reductionist, simplistic manner. From a UK perspective this can be demonstrated in a number of ways.

➤ Until comparatively recently statutory mental health services concentrated almost solely on the care of individuals with severe and enduring mental health problems. This situation arose out of research in the 1990s that indicated services were neglecting those in most need (i.e. individuals suffering from schizophrenia and major affective disorders).[10] The consequence of this was a government policy that directed services to concentrate on these individuals. This has led to situations where people with so-called less severe presentations have found it increasingly difficult to access mental health treatment. Although in recent times policy has become less rigid, it remains possible that diagnosis can determine the type of service that the individual can expect to receive – particularly where individuals may be thought to have a primary substance use problem. As many as 80% of such persons are believed to have mental health issues,[5] although certainly not all have schizophrenia or major affective disorder. Perversely, such individuals may also experience a limited welcome from substance use treatment agencies, who may consider that the underlying mental health issue is the primary problem. Consequently, the person may find themselves receiving, at best, serial treatment from different agencies or, at worst, no care at all. The problem has proved so acute that the UK government has had to issue direction on the matter. The guidance has outlined that where a person has a primary severe mental health problem, ambiguities about clinical responsibility should not be a barrier to treatment, stipulating that mental health services should take the lead. Where individuals have a primary substance use problem, substance use agencies may take the lead, but are entitled to expect collaboration from mental health services regarding any mental health concerns.[4]

➤ Within the UK there have existed, for some time, two somewhat recalcitrant debates about the merits of abstinence versus harm-reduction philosophy, and about the perceived harmfulness of alcohol compared with illegal substances. These debates have on occasion seemed quite fractious, leading to the dismissal of a senior government adviser in 2009 and the subsequent impression that policy is driven by political rather than scientific argument.[11] Government policy ultimately affects local funding as well as individual referring decisions. The limiting of choice and education and suppression of rational debate about treatment imperatives may serve to affect the type of substance use service one might receive. If a referrer has an undeveloped understanding of an individual's problem and appropriate treatment, the suitability of referrals can be rendered pure chance and a window of opportunity may be lost. The situation is further complicated where concurrent mental health–substance use problems occur. It has been contended that the traditional treatment preference by mental health professionals has been the promotion of abstinence to the exclusion of more pragmatic harm-reduction approaches; while abstinence may be considered preferable, it is acknowledged that the confrontational aspects sometimes employed are not always appropriate for people experiencing mental health–substance use problems.[8]

➤ As stated, mental health–substance use problems inevitably lead to a variety of deleterious consequences for the individual. The success of both mental health and substance use treatment is likely to prove limited unless due attention is given to these aspects. Fragmented family relationships, homelessness, physical and sexual abuse, unemployment, criminality and poor educational attainment may all underpin the development of mental health–substance use problems and are likely to increase in severity if remedial attention is not given. Therefore, the collaboration of specialist agencies outside of the immediate mental health and substance use arena should be sought and included within the overall package of care.

➤ Notions of risk can influence the care of individuals. In recent years, several homicides in the UK have gained a level of notoriety when it has been revealed that the perpetrators have had mental health–substance use problems.[3] Subsequent government policy has been influenced by such events and has inevitably had an impact on practice. In certain circumstances this may have led to a limitation of choice in the area of treatment, in that the guiding principle of 'motivation to change' becomes negligible when a community treatment order or similar statutory instrument is imposed to compel an individual into treatment. In such situations it may be argued that treatment agencies will be limited to a policing role. Alternatively it could be viewed that these circumstances provide opportunities for agencies to work together within a statutory framework to sustain community living for complex individuals who might otherwise face prolonged institutional care.[12]

➤ The legal and policy situation can be confusing and sometimes sends mixed messages to individuals and professionals alike. Under UK law the Misuse of Drugs Act 1971 sets out categories of classification for substances of misuse, and punishments for the possession and supply of such substances. Within the UK, alcohol is considered to have the most profound overall negative consequences for mental health. It has been argued that heavy alcohol consumption can lead to anxiety and depression, and it has been implicated in the 50 or so suicides that occur in Wales each year;[13] yet alcohol is not classified in the Act at all. This leaves us with policy initiatives that promote safer use by recommending arbitrary limits of alcohol consumption,[14] and laws that aim to curtail but not prohibit its purchase. The continued and socially acceptable use of alcohol by family and friends can be a powerful disincentive to individuals who have developed alcohol problems and need to address their own use.

As stated, within a Welsh context by far the most common and problematic substance of use is alcohol. In the substance use treatment field it has often been thought that the wider media obscured this issue in favour of sensationalist head-lines about the effects of illicit substances of use, although more recently the debate about the effects of binge drinking has become more noticeable. In the light of this it is pertinent to consider the process of assessment of individuals such as Tom, with mental health and alcohol use issues. Currently in Wales, assessment of mental health problems involves an initial Unified Assessment Process (UAP), and if an individual's problems are deemed severe enough the Care Programme Approach (CPA) will be implemented.[15] This involves completion of a structured document where different assessment domains are considered, the aim being completion of a comprehensive holistic assessment that follows the individual from service to service – thus avoiding repetitive questioning sometimes termed **serialised assess-ment**. The characteristics of this process are perhaps best described elsewhere, but what is apparent is that at a local level the notion that 'one assessment fits all' is an ambition yet to be realised, and when a person with mental health problems is referred to an alcohol agency further assessment will be required. Specifically, specialist agencies may find that the assessment domains in the UAP document are too generalist and do not contain enough detail to complete an accurate picture of an individual's alcohol problems, which is needed to inform the subsequent treat-ment process. Notwithstanding these limitations, the alcohol agency will need to be mindful that any additional assessment will still need to be viewed within the bigger picture that the UAP provides, and mental health professionals should be aware that even though alcohol agencies may well do more-specialised assessments, their own generalist assessment should continue to be as thorough as possible.

ASSESSMENT AND THE QUALITY OF BEING HUMAN
What is assessment?

Assessment is a continuous, cyclical process, beginning even before the professional and individual identify problematic issues. Once the provisional care plan is agreed, assessment continues throughout to ensure interventions and treatment are adjusted to meet the needs of the individual and family. However, there is usually a point at which the individual, family and professional sit down and systematically draw together information in order to decide on the exact nature of the problems and how best to move forward together.[16] The primary aim of assessment is threefold:

1 Information – gather accurate information (listening to the individual and family story) about:
   a   the person
   b   the family
   c   health problems
   d   associated problems.
2 Identify – factors associated with the health problems.
3 Coping strategies – explore strengths and weaknesses and the person's ability to cope with them; they play a pivotal role in the management of the health problems and other identified problems.[16]

Assessment involves two-way communication and enables the individual and family to express
➤ hopes
➤ fears
➤ expectations,

. . . and to receive information about the health problems, interventions, and treatment. This requires sensitivity and skill, which develops with experience and knowledge.

Why is assessment important?

Symptoms related to mental health–substance use problems do not exist in isolation. They cause other problems. Therefore, throughout the assessment the professional must consider the person-centred needs of the individual and family covering all aspects of the individual's life:
➤ physical
➤ psychological
➤ social
➤ emotional
➤ legal
➤ economical
➤ spiritual
➤ cultural.

While including highly clinical aspects, the professional's role is primarily to facilitate self-help. It is acknowledged that the individual is the expert in his/her care and needs[17] and the professional's role is to facilitate that expertise, to identify problems, and offer appropriate interventions and treatment, to achieve the individual's chosen goals. Thus, to plan care it is necessary to have good information about the individual's and family's:

➤ inclinations
➤ strengths
➤ abilities
➤ problems
➤ difficulties.

The intra- and interdisciplinary team may be involved with the individual and family (*see* Book 2, Chapters 11 and 12). Therefore, it is essential to identify each professional and the role each plays in the individual's life. This avoids overlap, enhances coordination and effective team working and relationships, and directs resources to the direct care of the individual.

Assessment questions are threefold:
1 What can I do for the individual and family?
2 What can the individual and family do for themselves?
3 How can I work alongside the individual and family to maintain their independence?

What should assessment include?
Every individual and family has a story to tell (*see* Book 1, Chapters 4, 6, 7, 8 and 9). Encourage the individual and family to each tell their story:

➤ using their own words
➤ in their own time.

This may be time-consuming but is time well spent. Without the person-centred picture, intervention and treatment is ineffective. Only when you – as the professional – have decided what information is needed can you clarify:

➤ why you need it
➤ what you will do with it.

During assessment ask yourself:
➤ what decisions do the individual, family and I have to make?
➤ what information is needed to aid the decision-making process?[16]

The process of assessment
Assessment should take place:
➤ in a safe place
➤ in a confidential environment
➤ with sensitivity towards issues of
  — race (*see* Chapter 5; Book 4, Chapters 3 and 4)
  — culture (*see* Chapter 5; Book 4, Chapters 3 and 4
  — gender (*see* Book 2, Chapter 14)

  — sexuality (*see* Book 2, Chapter 14)
  — religion and beliefs (*see* Book 2, Chapter 13)
  — age (*see* Book 3, Chapters 2, 3, 4, 5, 6 and 7)
  — legality (*see* Book 2, Chapter 15; Book 3, Chapter 14)
  — finance.

The way the assessment is conducted and information collected influences the rapport between the professional, individual and family, which in turn will affect the process of any interventions that follow.[16] Individuals most likely to engage are those who feel the professional is warm, accepting, understanding, knowledgeable and genuinely wants to work alongside them. Here lies the establishment of a therapeutic relationship and the quality of what it is to be human (*see* Book 4, Chapter 2).

Assessment tools
While helpful in aiding diagnosis or symptom severity, assessment tools do not take the place of a willingness to listen and the ability to understand the individual and family. Assessment tools can aid the flow and structure, and ensure specific information is obtained and/or measured. However, it is important to explain if you are going to write notes or complete an assessment tool, and to discuss the issue of confidentiality relating to information being shared.[18]

    Assessment tools can be disadvantageous, creating barriers among the individual, family and professional, and taking the focus away from the individual's identified needs or concerns. However, if they are completed with sensitivity, maintaining eye contact, they should not be intrusive to effective communication.

Primary factors of assessment
Assessment is:
➤ cyclical
➤ continuous
➤ ongoing
➤ detailed.

Eight primary factors can aid focus on points of assessment. By addressing these points a picture of the person's story develops that aids further interventions and assessment.
1 Right setting:
   a initial contact – building trust and therapeutic relationship
   b introduction – friendly, warm, social, negotiation.
2 Person's story:
   a understanding – the person's perspective
   b appreciation – of the person's emotional journey
   c judgement – requires good clinical judgement: the person may be unwell, tired and vulnerable
   d powerful and important – what the person has to say is integral to them and their ill health and problems.

3 What are the primary concerns:
   a explore – physical, psychological, spiritual, emotional, sexual, economic and social aspects
   b importance – what is important to the person?
   c symptoms – what is the most troublesome symptom?
   d directness – be direct when exploring symptoms.
4 What is the person's understanding of their:
   a ill health/problems – what does it mean to the person?
   b hopes
   c expectations
   d ideas
   e belief systems
   f support
   g worries.
5 Who is important to the person:
   a support from – who supports the person?
   b support to – is this person a carer?
6 Exploration of feelings:
   a ill health/problems – ask 'How does your ill health/problems make you feel?'
   b coping – ask 'What helps you cope?'
7 Listening:
   a attentive – listen to what is said and what is not said
   b silence – do not be afraid to use silence
   c touch – use appropriate touch to comfort and reassure
   d clarify – feed back and check to clarify and demonstrate your understanding and comprehension
   e summarise – bring together and clarify problems
   f explain – offer careful explanation of key points; explain in simple terms – for example, what is happening, what will happen next, medication, what the options are.
8 Sexuality:
   a under-acknowledged – often by the professional
   b expectations – individuals expect professionals to approach topics of sexuality
   c sensitivity – aim not to be intrusive; use a gentle, sensitive approach; demonstrate your openness to discuss; the person can choose whether or not to respond.

Skills used in assessment

There is a diversity of skills used during assessment. Each person is unique regardless of the lifestyle, religious beliefs or ethnic group and so on. It is important to believe in the person as an equal human being.[19] The professional should be aware of his/her own values to ensure a non-judgemental approach towards the individual and family. The way the assessment is conducted and information collected influences the rapport among the professional, the individual and family. This in turn affects the process of any treatment and interventions that follow.

Non-verbal communications

The use of non-verbal communication assists in demonstrating your interest and attention to the person. During a typical interaction between two people 33% of what is exchanged is verbal and 66% non-verbal. Therefore, it is imperative to:

➤ maintain a relaxed body posture
➤ maintain appropriate eye contact
➤ maintain physical openness – sitting with your face and body directly facing the individual
➤ lean slightly forward – without invading the individual's personal space
➤ use appropriate relaxed facial expressions, and occasional smiles
➤ nod your head in encouragement.

Active listening

Listening involves:

➤ receiving sounds
➤ accurately understanding their meaning.

To be listened to is therapeutic, without necessarily involving other interactions.[20]

➤ Be sensitive to vocal cues.
➤ Listening:
  – assists in creating a relationship – the individual feels heard and understood
  – enables the individual to begin to share her/his world with you
  – allows the individual sufficient time to talk and complete statements before asking further questions or making comments.

Silence

Silences may feel uncomfortable. The natural tendency is to break silences by speaking. However, it is important to consider the value of silence for both the individual and the professional. Advantages of silence include:

➤ silence may allow time for the individual and professional to collect their thoughts before continuing
➤ some individuals will inevitably be less communicative and require more encouragement to talk.

Encouragement

It is important to encourage communication; this might include:

➤ using **open** questions – 'How do you feel today?'
➤ offering verbal encouragement – 'Tell me more about that'
➤ keeping the focus on the individual's situation
➤ using your tone of voice to indicate interest.

Clarification of communication

Checking and feeding back your understanding of what has been said:

➤ demonstrates interest and clarifies meaning and intent
➤ facilitates the gathering and assimilation of detailed information.

Use questions that confirm the individual's meaning is understood – 'What do you mean by that?'

Empathy

Being alongside and demonstrating an understanding of the person's situation and experience is pivotal.

➤ Use statements to demonstrate an understanding from the person's perspective, assisting the individual to go into more depth.

➤ Try to be relaxed with natural and spontaneous responses.

➤ Be sensitive to the person's feelings but with awareness that we are unable to fully understand or appreciate another person's situation. We cannot **fix it**; we can only help the individual to explore it.

➤ The art of assessment is in the **listening**.

Issue to consider

Physical and psychological assessment for both the individual and the family is essential to ensure that appropriate levels of support, interventions and treatment can be offered. The information received at referral may be restricted to clinical findings, giving limited or no indication of the individual's main concerns and dilemmas.

Observations

SELF-ASSESSMENT EXERCISE 9.1

Time 10 minutes
What observation could you make while completing an assessment?

Observations are valuable not just of the individual's psychological health but also of the person's physical health. By taking into account the individual's general appearance, clothing, cleanliness, possible weight loss or gain, skin colour and clear symptoms, hallucinations, tremor, agitation, pain, breathlessness, the professional gains important supportive insight into the person's problems. With experience these observations are almost intuitive.

KEY TIP 9.1

Do not dismiss your intuitive feelings.
• They are there for a reason.
• They are telling you something.

Enquire about your observations. Ask further questions regarding physical and psychological symptoms. Establish specific details of symptoms and medication being taken on a regular basis, the effects of the prescribed medications and about other substances used. Ask about mobility limitations. The individual may not think this is important or may accidentally omit to tell you. Professionals require a knowledge based on symptom management and awareness to be able to interpret this information.

Checking

Check if symptoms restrict daily living – for example, work, social and leisure time. Experience will assist in alerting the professional to cues given by the individual – for example, 'I am not sleeping well.' This needs to be clarified and the problem established.

Clarify and enable understanding

Try to clarify the individual's and family's understanding of the prognosis and presenting problems. Enable the individual and family to talk about fears and feelings by encouraging open questions. The feelings may be expressed with anger about the situation, or open emotion with tears and obvious distress. However, do not assume you know what the anger is about – **ask!** For some it will be a relief to be able to talk openly to someone outside of the family, as they are reluctant to distress them further. Anxiety may be conveyed by:
➤ body language
➤ facial expression
➤ fidgeting with hand and fingers
➤ generalised restlessness.

The family will have their own concerns and fears. It is important to ensure they have an opportunity to express them, away from the individual if appropriate. Explore the usual family structure, their relationships with the individual and other family members. **Ask** about support available, or conflicts that may exist among family members. Be mindful that this type of information may not come to light until subsequent visits. Remember that **assessment is a continual, cyclical, ongoing process**.

Assessment: an ongoing process

The time taken to complete the assessment is determined by the responsiveness of the individual and the complexity of the situation. It is important that the assessment remain focused. However, time should be allowed for the individual to talk through their issues without feeling hurried.

Seek questions and contributions

Before concluding the assessment it is important to check if the individual or family have any further questions or concerns. At the end of each meeting with the individual and family:
➤ review the main problems as determined by the individual and family
➤ set priorities for these
➤ discuss an action plan
➤ discuss options and interventions
➤ encourage questions and clarification

➤ discuss with the individual and family the nature and frequency of further contacts
➤ ensure the individual and family know how to contact you
➤ plan for regular reviews
➤ reinforce any information given
➤ evaluate changes in the interventions
➤ liaise with other members of the intra- and interdisciplinary team.

Remember, some individuals will have problems that are long-standing; you may not be able to change these, other than offering emotional support and being there when needed. Inevitably, the individual's ill health and problems will cause distress for the individual, family and all their friends.

ASSESSMENT FOR MENTAL HEALTH–ALCOHOL PROBLEMS

Although the following will primarily consider the issues that arise in the assessment of people experiencing mental health–*alcohol* problems, the processes discussed have much in common with the assessment of individuals with mental health problems who use *other* substances.

The process of assessing

The process of assessing is complex. Professionals from different agencies may aim to meet the needs of individuals but there is often a gap or overlap of treatment. As discussed earlier, the care of individuals such as Tom may be coordinated by mental health services if they meet certain criteria. However, even if they do not, their mental health issues may still be serious enough to affect their ability to engage in substance use treatment. The National Treatment Agency (NTA) for Substance Misuse outlines an integrated model of care identifying four tiers of escalating complexity of assessment and interventions (*see* Box 9.1).[21] There needs to be an initial process to confirm and assess an individual's substance use and motivation. In primary care, an individual's substance use is often queried during routine consultations. There is debate about what happens with this information and unless there are significant physical health or social concerns it often remains on file with no further follow-up. There is also evidence to suggest under-reporting of alcohol use to professionals.[22,23]

BOX 9.1 Four-tier system[21]

Tier 1
This level mainly involves interventions from general healthcare and other services that are not specialist drug treatment services – for example, hospital emergency departments, pharmacies, general practitioners, antenatal wards and social care agencies. Tier 1 services offer facilities such as information and advice, screening for drug use and referral to specialist drug treatment services.

Tier 2
This is open-access drug treatment (such as drop-in services) that does not always

need a care plan. Tier 2 covers things like triage assessment, advice and information and harm reduction given by specialist drug treatment services.

Tier 3

This is drug treatment in the community with regular sessions to attend, undertaken as part of a care plan. Prescribing, structured day programmes and structured psychosocial interventions (counselling, therapy, and so forth) are always Tier 3. Advice, information and harm reduction can be Tier 3 if they are part of a care plan.

Tier 4

This is residential drug treatment – inpatient treatment and residential rehabilitation. Treatment should include arrangements for ongoing treatment or aftercare for individuals finishing treatment and returning to the community

To determine that the most appropriate treatment options are explored it is essential to ascertain the individual's drinking levels, patterns and usage, identifying whether their use is harmful or if there is evidence of dependence and addiction. Tom's case shows how alcohol use can slowly increase and often, due to its social acceptance, the effects can be obscured, especially if it is used as a coping mechanism or a means to self-medicate mental health symptoms. The individual's physical, psychological and social well-being also need to be assessed, as does the impact on others of the person's drinking (family members, friends, children and the wider community). It is also necessary to assess the person's motivation and readiness to change their substance use.[24] An informal history and examination may miss many people who have an alcohol problem.

Alcohol is believed to have the most negative overall consequences for mental health and, as with Tom, it can lead to many deleterious psychosocial consequences. Some definitions for alcohol use are listed in Box 9.2.[25]

BOX 9.2 UK definitions used by the models of care for people experiencing alcohol problems[25]

- **Low risk** – sensible drinking: up to 21 units per week for men and 14 units per week for women
- **Hazardous drinking** – up to 50 units per week for men and 35 units for women
- **Harmful drinking** – over 50 units per week for men and over 35 units for women
- **Moderately dependent** – includes psychological dependence and excess use affecting an individual's health and social functioning
- **Severely dependent** – associated with physical dependence and withdrawal symptoms upon cessation of alcohol

Professionals who identify significant alcohol use may refer individuals to specialist services or provide brief interventions and advice themselves. The prerequisite of partnership working with the individual is to ensure that the most appropriate and acceptable treatment options have been explored. Coordination among agencies and services is important to ensure that people do not fall through the service provision net (*see* Book 2, Chapters 11 and 12). The assessment of risk to self, others and children is an ongoing process and is an integral element of assessment at all levels.[5]

Disorganised treatment providers are likely to create poor outcomes; once a poor impression is experienced by the individual it may be difficult to overcome and the impact it has is often carried on throughout treatment.[26] The Models of Care for Alcohol Misusers[25] recognises the wide range of alcohol-related problems and has used the World Health Organization international classification of diseases (ICD)[27] to recommend that commissioners provide tiers of intensifying treatment interventions. Treatment should be organised and provided in a stepped care arrangement, whereby individuals are offered the least intrusive treatment options first, before reviewing the need for more comprehensive treatment.[22]

Assessment

The assessment process itself is an effective intervention for reducing the level of alcohol consumption in people drinking above the recommended limits, by changing their perception of their problem and highlighting their commitment to change. Assessment to obtain information about the person and their alcohol problem requires skill, and workers need to provide a non-confrontational, empathic and committed approach, involving family and carers wherever possible. Assessment varies in its depth and level of detail depending on the purpose and anticipated outcome of the assessment process.

Targeted screening tools (*see* Chapter 8) and validated questionnaires provide a higher rate of detection of an alcohol problem and can be used during general health checks and consultations in primary care (*see* Box 9.1 – Tier 1). The use of clinical questionnaires to aid understanding of alcohol use is well established in certain settings, although it can be difficult to ascertain what questionnaires are used and how services evaluate their use. Several tools are available for identification and brief advice including a variety of training tools. However, it should be stressed that tools are an aid and not a replacement for robust one-to-one assessment. At present, the UK government does not provide definitive guidance on which tools to use as this depends on alcohol harm-reduction intervention activity at a local level.[28] Questionnaires that have been validated include:

➤ Fast Alcohol Screening Test (FAST) specifically for use within emergency departments and medical settings to quickly assess for alcohol use. It consists of four questions aimed at identifying hazardous or harmful drinking as well as alcohol-related harm and dependence.
➤ Cut down, Annoyed, Guilty and Eye-opener (CAGE)
➤ Michigan Alcoholism Screening Test (MAST)
➤ Alcohol Use Disorder Identification Test (AUDIT) – advocated by the World Health Organization, AUDIT is recognised as the most effective screening tool for the identification of alcohol problems. The tool provides clear guidance on recommended intensity of intervention.

➤ Tolerance, Annoyed, Cut down, Eye-opener (T-ACE) – validated to use during pregnancy
➤ Tolerance, Worried, Eye-opener, Amnesia, Cut down (TWEAK).[25,29–31]

The assessment process has three recognised levels – screening, triage, comprehensive.

1 Screening

Screening is a brief process, most likely to be completed in a generic setting, the focus being to determine whether an alcohol problem exists and whether to refer to alcohol treatment services. Screening assessment may incorporate or be followed by a brief intervention. It may also include:
➤ identification of coexisting problems – for example, physical, psychological or social
➤ identification of immediate risk – for example, self-harm, physical health, self-neglect, suicide risk, harm to others (including children and vulnerable adults), pregnancy, domestic violence, harm to staff and risk of drinking and driving
➤ an assessment of the subsequent urgency of referral.

2 Triage

Triage or initial assessment will take place when an individual first makes contact with a specialist alcohol service. This assessment should not be as in-depth as a comprehensive assessment although it should cover all domains. It provides a fuller assessment than screening; it should fit into the care pathway of the individual and should provide an initial care plan outlining treatment options. It should also include an assessment of an individual's motivation to engage in treatment, current risk factors and the urgency of need. To determine the intervention or tier of service best suited to the individual it is important to consider the following:
➤ an overview of alcohol and drug use, including frequency and quantity of current and past use
➤ indicators of dependence (completed AUDIT)
➤ presenting physical and mental health issues
➤ presenting social issues
➤ treatment history including episodes of non-engagement
➤ criminal justice involvement
➤ measure of motivation and readiness to change
➤ the individual's preferred treatment options
➤ risk assessment
➤ priority status.

3 Comprehensive

Comprehensive assessment may be completed by one or more members of the intra- and interdisciplinary team due to the complex nature of an individual's presentation. Comprehensive assessments highlight individuals who may
➤ require structured and/or intensive intervention

➤ have significant coexisting physical and mental health problems
➤ have a significant level of risk of harm to self and/or others
➤ be in contact with multiple service providers
➤ have a history of disengagement from alcohol treatment services
➤ be pregnant or have children who may be at risk.

A comprehensive assessment provides the individual and worker with information that will contribute to the development of a care plan. Individuals may present with a range of problems for which they require additional help, and professionals should be mindful of the following issues:

➤ Measurements of alcohol in blood, urine or breath are useful for identifying acute alcohol levels. Alcohol-related disorders such as liver disease could appear in people without alcohol dependence. Thus, the role of clinical questionnaires in concurrence with biomarkers is seen as best practice to determine evidence of low-to-moderate alcohol use and harmful-to-hazardous use. There is evidence to support the use of biomarkers and there appears to be consensus that carbohydrate-deficient transferrin is considered to be the more *specific* marker and gamma-glutamyl transferase the more *sensitive* marker of chronic alcohol use.[32]

➤ The need for professionals to be knowledgeable about local services is paramount, as some individuals require information or referral to other agencies. Sometimes the professional may decide that a straightforward treatment is indicated, such as detoxification, but the individual may dispute this and desire other, unrealistic options. The assessment process therefore requires the professional to have a degree of skill in motivational interviewing and solution focused work, to help address the individual's concerns prior to the recommended treatment (*see* Chapters 10, 11 and 12; Book 4, Chapters 6–9).[22]

➤ The screening and assessment of alcohol in primary care has significant validation for timely interventions in people with alcohol use problems. Identifying individuals in primary care who are likely to gain from brief interventions will also assist in achieving targets set out in the UK's harm-reduction strategy,[33] although primary care professionals may be concerned about the time spent on integrating alcohol screening into their consultations.

➤ Detailed comprehensive assessment forms can be multifaceted, not practical, and get in the way of building a rapport with the individual. Over-complicated assessment processes may cause an increase in dropout rates and it should be remembered that clinical tools are there to help, not hinder, the assessment process.[34]

Intra- and interdisciplinary team working

Other services and agencies that may also be actively involved with individuals such as Tom include:

➤ social care and housing teams
➤ social services
➤ community mental health teams (CMHTs)

➤ youth services
➤ probation/police
➤ voluntary organisations
➤ employment and training services
➤ general practitioners
➤ general hospitals
➤ specialist liver units (*see* Book 2, Chapters 11 and 12).[14]

It is essential that there are clear lines of communication among the tiers of treatment intervention to help progress appropriate referrals. With integrated care planning, as well as the use of joint interagency protocols, the care coordination of individuals being seen by the most appropriate services will inevitably improve the standards of care.

Assessing for interventions

It is essential to differentiate between *dependence* and *addiction*. An individual's level of dependence may require medical interventions such as detoxification, while their addiction requires the assessor to evaluate the consequences of use across every facet of the individual's life. Once there is clear understanding and differences highlighted it is important to tailor the response to the needs of the *individual* and not the service.[22]

Within the assessment framework there are domains that need to be explored systematically to ensure that the right treatment is provided at the right time by the right service.[25] There is no interpretative formation that can help the assessor; the assessment process may be seen as an exercise in relevance that needs to be reviewed constantly.

During the assessment process the core issues in each *domain* emphasise what keeps and maintains the individual's problematic alcohol use; the *key indicators* outline the dissonance in social functioning across the life of the individual. Domains are as follows:
➤ alcohol and drug use
➤ social functioning – for example, employment, housing, finances, family, social life
➤ sexuality
➤ spirituality
➤ criminal justice involvement
➤ physical and mental health.[25]

During the assessment process, the individual has a wealth of knowledge about how their alcohol use affects the domains; the majority of which come from earlier treatment interventions. The need to review care plans in line with the concerns in each of the domains provides consistency and focus for the individual and professional. The skills of the professional should include the ability to see the bigger picture and explore discrepancies within the individual's story. During assessment it is essential that there is recognition of how difficult it may be for the individual to disclose personal issues. The professional will need to provide information about ways to change behaviour, identify clear treatment pathways and help in accessing other services if required.

The Pembrokeshire (Wales) model

In March 2007, three separate agencies provided alcohol assessment and treatment services in the region: the local county council, the National Health Service (NHS) and a voluntary organisation. All three services had an open referral system. Individuals were seen and assessed by any of these services and sometimes were seen by all of them. There was a scattergun approach for referring individuals to alcohol services from other agencies such as probation, housing support, voluntary sector providers and general practitioners. Individuals would self-refer and drift among services; disengagement with treatment was common. Individuals with chaotic alcohol use and complex issues would at times have unplanned admissions to the local general hospital with alcohol-related problems such as acute intoxication and severe withdrawals. Referrals from CMHTs to alcohol services included individuals who were difficult to engage due to their chaotic lifestyle and alcohol use, and those who experienced complications following sudden cessation from alcohol.

Professionals within each service had good informal relationships, often sharing information and referring to one another's service on an individual basis. Professionals from all three services provided a range of assessments and interventions such as brief interventions, relapse prevention, family support, harm reduction and home detoxifications. The professional mix comprised nurses, social workers, project workers, support workers and a consultant psychiatrist in substance use. There was a willingness to explore new ways of working to ease pressure on caseloads and reduce waiting lists; collaboratively the three services implemented a pilot project with an innovative model of working in the community. The concept was based on a stepped care model in line with the best practice described in this chapter. This approach uses an integrated model of care with four tiers of assessment and interventions, underpinned by working in partnership with the individual to formulate the most appropriate treatment options. Individuals are offered the least intrusive treatment options first, before reviewing the need for more comprehensive treatment.

While the voluntary organisation provided a Tier 2 service and the statutory services provided Tier 3 and Tier 4 services, at times the eligibility criteria were blurred between these agencies (*see* Box 9.1). Following implementation of the model, referrals are filtered through the Tier 2 service, and receive an initial assessment, normally within ten days. These are then discussed at the allocation meeting and forwarded to the most appropriate service, joint assessments being common due to the complexities of this individual group. There are now very clear treatment pathways for individuals, ensuring they have the right treatment at the right time by the right service. There has been a significant change in working relationships with the CMHTs and criminal justice service to ensure that individuals do not slip through the net due to their vulnerable presentation. Joint working has allowed Pembrokeshire individuals experiencing a problem with alcohol to receive a consistent, quality and seamless approach to their needs. It has also formalised working relationships and increased professional motivation and enthusiasm. The service

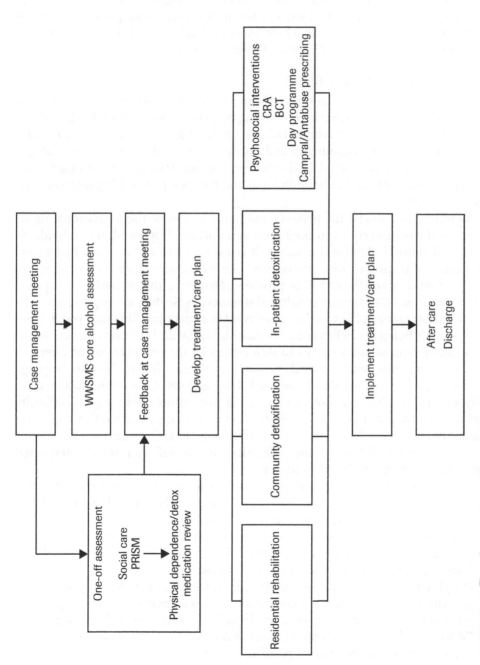

FIGURE 9.1 Flowchart treatment journey

is now collectively known as 'Pembrokeshire Alcohol Services' and there is a positive spirit about team working. This model of working has also been implemented in neighbouring localities and appears to be working well. The flowchart (*see* Figure 9.1) shows the treatment journey for the individual with possible treatment interventions after assessment in a Tier 3 service. Each tier will also have their own care pathway for specific treatment and interventions.

CULTURAL CONSIDERATIONS[35]

Any individual – regardless of race, culture, colour, creed, social and/or economic status – has the right to expect and receive appropriate interventions, treatment and care. For some, the lack of adequate cultural knowledge will prevent proper interactions taking place in a meaningful and purposeful way. The issue of transcultural health and social care is broad. In this section, we look at some of the problems and difficulties encountered by the individual and family when seeking interventions and treatment.

As well as addressing the person's and family's history, the professional needs to assess the issues related to migration and culture. If ignored, the individual's racial and cultural identity is rebuffed. It is a mistake to assume that, by treating an individual from an ethnic minority as one would any other person, adequate interventions and treatment will be provided. Moreover, the professional may deal with the individual and family as **cultural stereotypes**. Such an approach ignores the social and interpersonal factors that are relevant in assessment. This often results from professionals being overwhelmed by unfamiliar racial and cultural characteristics.

Another difficult area relates to differences in the presentation of physical, psychological, emotional, spiritual and social problems. Where there are language difficulties, an interpreter should be used. The interpreter, however, must be carefully selected. If she/he is not from a caring profession, there may be difficulty explaining information or asking questions in a meaningful way; if the interpreter is a member of the individual's family, this can lead to embarrassment.

Some examples follow of how references and beliefs can be misinterpreted through lack of knowledge of cultural issues.

➤ When a person of Pakistan origin refers to him/herself as being 'royal', he/she is not necessarily deluded; it means simply that he/she comes from a wealthy family. This is not a grandiose delusion in cultural terms.

➤ 'The good Lord is talking to me' is an expression often used by Afro-Caribbean people of religious background. This can be misconstrued as the individual experiencing auditory hallucinations.

➤ Peoples of Asian, East Indian and African descent can have what appears to be bruising that is common among darker-skinned persons. For example, what appears to be bruising on a child's body or on the individual can be 'Mongolian blue spot'. Do not to jump to conclusions without adequate exploration and assessment of possible concerns.

Building a rapport requires time, patience, tolerance and perseverance. The individual and/or family may be reluctant to allow a cultural outsider to get too close. The style of questioning adopted by Western society often does not fit the conceptual models used in other cultures. The professional who insists on using this style of questioning may lose credibility in that he/she may be perceived as ignorant. This makes it difficult to facilitate participation and involvement in intervention and treatment. Conversely, members of other cultures often expect the professional to have all the answers.

Interventions and treatment should be as free from trauma as possible. The individual and family from a minority culture are often disadvantaged in a system designed for white Europeans. To conclude this section, there follows a list of **'do's** and **'do not's** (Box 9.3), that applies to all cultures. The list is not exhaustive; it can be used as a reference when working with individuals from any culture.

BOX 9.3 Cultural considerations – 'do's and 'do not's[35]

Name
- Do not:
  - use Western titles (e.g. Mr, Miss, Ms, Mrs)
  - ask non-Christians for a Christian name.
- Do:
  - ask for family name or first name
  - ask what name the person prefers you use (e.g. Mr or Miss or first name)
  - use the chosen form of address
  - avoid repetition in clinical notes; find out the correct name first rather than misuse several different names.

Language
- Do not:
  - assume that all ethnic groups speak English
  - assume that all minority ethnic groups do not speak English
  - use the family to interpret intimate questions
  - use the family to break bad news; she/he may avoid the issue if it is believed to be too stressful for the individual.
- Do:
  - avoid making assumptions by using accurate assessment procedures
  - use an interpreter who understands medical terminology; this will avoid stress for the interpreter, individual and family and avoid misinterpretation.

Religion
- Do not:
  - generalise about the individual's or family's religion
  - mistake religious objects or symbols for jewellery.
- Do:
  - remember that for Buddhist, Christian, Jewish, Sikh, Hindu and Muslim people religion may be an integral part of daily life
  - avoid incorrect assumptions; find out the different beliefs and approaches
  - record clearly and make a note of the individual's or family's wish to see or have a religious representative present

— ask the family if the individual is not able to relay this to you
— remember that many Eastern religions fast on certain days; pray at certain times; wear religious objects and symbols
— check if interventions or treatments will compromise any religious beliefs
— inform the individual and family of any interventions or treatments, before commencing, to check religious beliefs
— check religious observations with the individual and family
— consult religious advisers or teachers to gain permission and/or to obtain exemption to allow procedures to take place; ensure she/he explains this to the individual and family.

Diet

- Do not:
  — give Jewish or Muslim people pork or pork products
- Do:
  — make sure that other meat offered to Muslim people has been religiously slaughtered by the Halal method (natural slaughter)
  — remember that not all Jewish people eat Kosher food (specially prepared to be pure)
  — remember not all Muslim people eat Halal meat
  — consult the individual and family about any dietary preferences
  — remember that meal times are family occasions in Eastern cultures; matters relating to family are often discussed then
  — remember that being taken out of a close family environment can be frightening and cause loneliness, which may in turn cause loss of appetite
  — invite the family to bring food and join in meal times, if at all possible; if this is not practicable, explain why.

Personal hygiene

- Do:
  — remember that to Sikh, Hindu and Muslim people, washing in still water is considered unclean
  — supply the individual with a jug of water and bowl and/or running tap and empty washbasin to allow hand, face and body washing
  — make exceptions if the individual is dependent
  — remember that Muslim people use the right hand for eating and preparing food, and the left hand for self-cleaning and other procedures; anyone unable to do this because of injury or health reasons will need counselling and discussion relating to ways of surmounting this problem (it may be useful to supply plastic gloves).

Modesty

- Do not:
  — compromise the individual's dignity and modesty.
- Do:
  — remember that to expose the female body to a male will cause distress in certain cultures, especially if the individual is in purdah (the duration of menstruation)

 — offer separate bays in mixed bedded wards or, if possible, a single room, especially if the person is in purdah
 — remember that hospital gowns expose more than they cover and therefore are often unacceptable
 — avoid exposure of arms and legs; add additional covering to protect modesty.

Skin and hair
* Do:
  — remember that Afro-Caribbean people's hair may be brittle or dry; add moisturiser or oil to the scalp and comb regularly
  — remember to ask the individual what she/he uses for skin moisturiser
  — remember that dark-skinned people are prone to keloid scarring (hyperkeratinisation); invasive treatment will cause excessive pigmented scarring
  — remember to inject or undertake invasive procedures at a site that will avoid disfigurement if possible.

Hospital procedures
* Do not:
  — give Jehovah's Witness people blood transfusions
  — give Muslim, Jewish and vegetarian people iron injections derived from pigs
  — give insulin of bovine origin to Hindu and Sikh people
  — give insulin of porcine origin to Jewish or Muslim people.
* Do:
  — give careful thought to procedures and routines before commencing them
  — remember that discussion of elimination or other intimate issues may be culturally offensive
  — approach all individuals sensitively; ensure privacy and maintain the individual's right to self-respect
  — remember that some medications, interventions and treatments may be taboo for some religious groups
  — remember that some medications have an alcohol base, which may be forbidden in some cultural groups
  — remember that individuals with alcohol problems may wish to avoid alcohol-based preparations
  — be aware of all preparations likely to contain potentially taboo or offensive ingredients.

Visiting
* Do:
  — remember that limiting visiting to two people may cause distress in extended family cultures
  — remember West Indian, Asian and Middle Eastern families like to visit as a family
  — remember that family may include children, uncles, aunts, grandchildren, parents and grandparents

— compromise over visiting, and numbers of visitors per individual, if possible
— remember that open visiting is more accommodating
— allow the family to participate in the individual's care.

Pain myths
- Do not:
  — believe that people from different races have a low pain threshold; this is incorrect; for example:
    (i) Japanese people may smile or laugh when in pain, thus avoiding loss of face
    (ii) Anglo-Saxon people may be sullen and withdrawn, portraying the 'stiff-upper-lip' image
    (iii) Eastern Europeans, Greeks and Italian people express pain vocally and freely.
- Do:
  — remember that every individual has a different level of pain tolerance, regardless of race, colour or creed.

Death and bereavement
- Do not:
  — deny a person the right to participate in last offices as this will increase the pain already being expressed and may slow down the grieving process.
- Do:
  — involve the individual and family in care
  — remember that Eastern European cultures like to take an active part in the care of the dying relative, especially last offices
  — remember that in certain cultures, custom and practice will need to be followed if the individual is to proceed along the continuum of life following his/her earthly death
  — ensure you are fully conversant with specific cultural requirements for death, bereavement and last offices
  — negotiate to minimise anxiety and allow some participation when the family's wishes come into conflict with hospital policies and procedures – this will assist the grieving process
  — compromise; the individual and family have only one chance to say their goodbyes.

CONCLUSION

Although this chapter has primarily considered the contemporary issues that arise in the assessment of people with mental health and *alcohol* difficulties, the processes discussed have much in common with the assessment of individuals with mental health–*substance use* problems. It has been shown that mental health–substance use issues are often complex, and solutions to the problem need to take into account a wide range of psychosocial factors as well as the immediate treatment issues. The authors show how assessment of these problems can be accomplished, mindful that this needs to take place within a broader collaborative framework where different helping agencies will all have their own agendas. Assessment of an individual's problems can never be truly complete. As a person negotiates a treatment pathway changing needs will occur. Resolution of alcohol problems may reveal underlying difficulties that were not initially apparent; alternatively, improvement in presentation may enable the individual to move on in terms of occupation, housing and re-establishing old relationships. Mental health–substance use issues are complex and difficulties in treatment should be anticipated. Yet, problems can be overcome by effective collaboration among all professionals and services, and this can lead to optimism that individuals in treatment can progress to lead productive and fulfilling lives.

The nature of assessment must vary to suite the circumstances of the individual and family. Although the prime focus will be the ill health and its associated problems, this needs to be understood in context with the individual's life, beliefs and values. Rather than seeing assessment as the professional collecting information and forming clinical judgements, it is more accurate to think of the individual, family and professional jointly assessing the problems and considering possible solutions.

As professionals working in mental health–substance use care, we are privileged to encounter people at a distressing time in their lives. This requires a person-centred approach, using sensitivity and skills to complete an assessment before being able to initiate an action plan and appropriate interventions and treatment.

ACKNOWLEDGEMENT

The authors wish to express their sincere thanks to: Brooks M. Assessment in palliative care. In: Cooper J, editor. *Stepping into Palliative Care 2: care and practice.* 2nd ed. Oxford and USA: Radcliffe Publishing; 2006. (© Cooper J) for permitting the modifications and amendments to the chapter in the section headed: 'Assessment and the quality of being human'. Also to: Cooper DB. Transcultural issues and approaches. In: Wright H, Giddey M, editors. *Mental Health Nursing: from first principle to professional practice.* London: Chapman & Hall; 1992. (© Cooper DB) for permitting the modification and amendments to the chapter in the section headed 'Cultural considerations'.

REFERENCES

1 Menezes PR, Johnson S, Thornicroft G, *et al.* Drug and alcohol problems among individuals with severe mental illness in south London. *British Journal of Psychiatry.* 1996; **168**: 612–9.

2 Weaver T, Madden P, Charles V, *et al.* Comorbidity of substance misuse and mental illness in community mental health and substance misuse services. *British Journal of Psychiatry.* 2003; **183**: 304–13.

3 University of Manchester. *Five Year Report of the National Confidential Inquiry into Suicide and Homicide by People with Mental Illness.* 2006. Available at: www.medicine.manchester.ac.uk/psychiatry/research/suicide/prevention/nci/reports/avoidabledeathsfullreport.pdf (accessed 24 January 2011).

4 Welsh Assembly Government. *A Service Framework to Meet the Needs of People with a Co-occurring Substance Misuse and Mental Health Problem.* 2007. Available at: www.wales.nhs.uk/documents/CooccurringENGLISHFINAL.pdf (accessed 5 October 2010).

5 Department of Health. *Mental Health Policy Implementation Guide: dual diagnosis good practice guide*. 2002. Available at: www.dh.gov.uk/prod_consum_dh/groups/dh_digital assets/@dh/@en/documents/digitalasset/dh_4060435.pdf (accessed 5 October 2010).

6 Department of Health. *Dual Diagnosis in Mental Health Inpatient and Day Hospital Settings: guidance on the assessment and management of patients in mental health inpatient and day hospital settings who have mental ill-health and substance use problems*. 2006. Available at: www.dh.gov.uk/prod_consum_dh/groups/dh_digitalassets/@dh/@en/documents/digital asset/dh_062652.pdf (accessed 5 October 2010).

7 Coombes L, Wratten A. The lived experience of community mental health nurses working with people who have dual diagnosis: a phenomenological study. *Journal of Psychiatric and Mental Health Nursing*. 2007; **14**: 382–92.

8 Phillips P, Labrow J. Dual diagnosis: does harm reduction have a role? *International Journal of Drug Policy*. 2000; **11**: 279–83.

9 Graham HL. Implementing integrated treatment for co-existing substance use and severe mental health problems in assertive outreach teams: training issues. *Drug and Alcohol Review*. 2004; **23**: 463–70.

10 Gournay K. The changing face of psychiatric nursing: revisiting mental health nursing. *Advances in Psychiatric Treatment*. 2005; **11**: 6–11.

11 Lister S. *Professor David Nutt Attacks Ministers over 'Failure' on Alcohol*. 2009. Available at: www.timesonline.co.uk/tol/news/politics/article6903660.ece (accessed 5 October 2010).

12 Adams M, Evans L. Mental health and substance use. In: National forensic nurses' research and development group: Kettles A, Woods P, Byrt R, editors. *Forensic Mental Health Nursing: capabilities, roles and responsibilities*. London: Quay Books; 2008. pp. 247–58.

13 National Public Health Service for Wales. *Alcohol and Health in Wales: a major public health issue*. Cardiff: Cardiff University: 2006. Available at: www2.nphs.wales.nhs. uk:8080/VulnerableAdultsDocs.nsf/Public/C866F51E7F03DB32802571AA002F6081/ $File/ATT6QLZ1.doc (accessed 5 October 2010).

14 Department of Health. *Alcohol Advice*. London: DOH; 2009. Available at: http://web archive.nationalarchives.gov.uk/+/www.dh.gov.uk/en/Publichealth/Healthimprovement/ Alcoholmisuse/DH_085385 (accessed 6 February 2011).

15 Welsh Assembly Government. *Adult Mental Health Services: raising the standard. the revised adult mental health national service framework and an action plan for Wales*. Cardiff: 2005. Available at: www.wales.nhs.uk/documents/WebsiteEnglishNSFandActionPlan.pdf (accessed 5 October 2010).

16 Mason P. Essential of assessment. In: Cooper DB, editor. *Alcohol Use*. Oxford, Radcliffe Publishing; 2000. pp. 161–71.

17 Department of Health. *The Expert Patient: a new approach to chronic disease management in the 21st century*. London: Stationery Office; 2001.

18 Faulkner A, Maguire P. *Talking to Cancer Patients and Their Relatives*. Oxford: Oxford University Press; 1994.

19 Davies B, Oberle K. Dimensions of the supportive role of the nurse in palliative care. *Oncology Nursing Forum*. 1990; **17**: 87–94.

20 Nelson-Jones R. *Practical Counselling and Helping Skills*. 2nd ed. London: Cassell; 1988.

21 National Treatment Agency for Substance Misuse. *Explaining the Tier System*. London, NTA. Available at: http://nta.shared.hosting.zen.co.uk/about_treatment/the_tier_system. aspx (accessed 5 October 2010).

22 Harris P. *Empathy for the Devil: how to help people overcome drugs and alcohol problems*. Lyme Regis: Russell House Publishing; 2007.

23 Alcohol Concern. Primary Concern: Special Conference Edition. *PCAIS Newsletter.* 4; Spring 2002. London: Alcohol Concern.

24 Prochaska JO, DiClemente CC. The transtheoretical approach. In: Norcross JC, Goldfried MR, editors. *Handbook of Psychotherapy Integration.* 2nd ed. New York: Oxford University Press; 2005. pp. 147–71.

25 Department of Health. *Models of Care for Alcohol Misusers (MoCAM).* London: DOH; 2006. Available at: www.dh.gov.uk/prod_consum_dh/groups/dh_digitalassets/@dh/@en/documents/digitalasset/dh_4136809.pdf (accessed 5 October 2010).

26 Raistrick D, Heather N, Godfrey C. *Review of the Effectiveness of Treatment for Alcohol Problems.* London: NTA; 2006. Available at: www.nta.nhs.uk/publications/documents/nta_review_of_the_effectiveness_of_treatment_for_alcohol_problems_fullreport_2006_alcohol2.pdf (accessed 5 October 2010).

27 World Health Organization. *Mental and Behavioural Disorders Due to Psychoactive Substance Use.* 2007. Available at: http://apps.who.int/classifications/apps/icd/icd10online/ (accessed 5 October 2010).

28 Department of Health. *Local Routes: guidance for developing alcohol treatment pathways.* London: DOH; 2009. Available at: www.dh.gov.uk/prod_consum_dh/groups/dh_digital assets/documents/digitalasset/dh_110422.pdf (accessed 5 October 2010).

29 Trenoweth S, Tobutt C. Assessing alcohol use and misuse in primary care. In: Martin C, editor. *Identification and Treatment of Alcohol Dependency.* Keswick: M&K Publishing; 2008. pp. 15–24.

30 Chan AW, Pristach EA, Welte JW, *et al.* Use of the TWEAK test in screening for alcoholism/heavy drinking in three populations. *Alcoholism: Clinical and Experimental Research.* 1993; **17**: 1188–92.

31 Chang G, Wilkins-Haug L, Berman S, *et al.* The TWEAK: application in a prenatal setting. *Journal of Studies on Alcohol.* 1999; **60**: 306–9.

32 SriRajaskanthan R, Preedy VR. Diagnosis and management of alcoholic liver disease. In: Martin C, editor. *Identification and Treatment of Alcohol Dependency.* Keswick: M&K Publishing; 2008. pp. 55–66.

33 Department of Health, Home Office, Department for Education and Skills, Department for Culture, Media and Sport. *Safe. Sensible. Social: the next steps in the National Alcohol Strategy.* London: DOH; 2007. Available at: www.dh.gov.uk/prod_consum_dh/groups/dh_digitalassets/@dh/@en/documents/digitalasset/dh_075219.pdf (accessed 5 October 2010).

34 Gossop M. *Drug Addiction and Its Treatment.* London: Oxford University Press; 2003.

35 Cooper DB. Transcultural issues and approaches. In: Wright H, Giddey M, editors. *Mental Health Nursing: from first principles to professional practice.* London: Chapman & Hall; 1993. pp. 191–201.

TO LEARN MORE

- Cooper DB. *Alcohol Home Detoxification and Assessment.* Oxford: Radcliffe Publishing; 1994.
- Cooper DB, editor. *Alcohol Use.* Oxford: Radcliffe Publishing; 2000.
- Rassool GH, editor. *Dual Diagnosis Nursing.* Oxford: Blackwell; 2006.
- Adams M. Comorbidity of mental health and substance misuse problems: a review of workers' reported attitudes and perceptions. *Journal of Psychiatric and Mental Health Nursing.* 2008; **15**: 101–8.

CHAPTER 10

Brief intervention

Karl V Robins and David A Hingley

INTRODUCTION

When working with people with complex needs – that is, with 'coexisting mental health and substance misuse problems'[1] – traditional, orthodox treatment approaches are based around practitioners establishing the chronology of presenting problems, and determining whether they require independent treatment or whether treating one will help alleviate the other. Gaining a person-centred picture of the individual's current lifestyle, domestic arrangements and historical factors is seen as fundamental.

People with added stress or the beginnings of a mental illness sometimes try to escape their problems and symptoms by using substances. Often this makes the initial 'problem' worse. Traditional helping approaches concentrate on the 'problem' and emphasise the need to understand it and to recognise where it comes from in order to begin to do something about it. This assumes that problems and symptoms are at the centre of the person's life and, thus, are the focus for interventions. An alternative approach is solution focused brief therapy (SFBT).

THE SOLUTION FOCUSED APPROACH

In solution focused work, emphasis is on a future where the 'problem' either does not exist or is less intrusive, and on the times in the past and present when the 'problematic' events have not occurred or have not been as prominent. The description of a problem-free time provides the individual with clues and ideas about how to change and regain control over their life.

The future is created and negotiated, and not a slave of the past events in a person's life; therefore, in spite of past traumatic events, a person can negotiate and implement many useful steps that are likely to lead him/her to a more satisfying life.[2]

This approach considers:

➤ That the person is **not** the problem; the problem is the problem and occurs in interactions between people. The person 'is simply *in* the problem or under its influence.'[3]

➤ There is no such thing as a perfect problem; there are 'circumstances in which the stated problem
   − does not occur

- — occurs less often or less intensely
- — is in some way different from its regular state.'[4]
- ➤ That we all have the ability to find our own solutions to the difficulties that we encounter.
- ➤ That the future is dynamic and subject to change. Change is inevitable and constantly occurs. Change is so much a part of living that people cannot prevent themselves from changing.[5]
- ➤ That small changes can begin a process of making a difference, and problems that initially may appear to be fairly complex do not necessarily require complex solutions.[6]

Because of the difficulties encountered by people with complex needs, focusing on solutions and helpful strategies is often a difficult task. However, an individual's own solution is more likely to fit their particular situation and, therefore, is more likely to be implemented and maintained.

No single solution fits everyone and every situation; therefore, identifying what works for each individual is important. The approach focuses on exploring possibilities and increasing choices, rather than changing behaviours. In order for this to happen, the practitioner takes on '*a curious, "unknowing" stance with the individual, letting him or her become the expert on the presenting problem*.'[7]

SOLUTION FOCUSED BRIEF THERAPY: BASIC PREMISES

> If it ain't broke, don't fix it.
> Find out what works and do more of it.
> If it doesn't work, do something different.[8]

McFarland[9] comments that the practitioner should be concerned only with what the individual actively presents as the problem (and not what the practitioner believes is the problem). When the therapist and the person discover a time (or times) when the problem is not occurring, then a solution has probably been discovered and the individual needs to concentrate more on this. If something does not work, it is to be rigorously avoided. Doing something else, something 'different', becomes a focus for the person in coping with their life situations. Solution focused practitioners distinguish between problems and life situations or limitations.

THE LANGUAGE OF SOLUTION FOCUSED THERAPY

If we want to go somewhere, the questions that we ask ourselves focus on the future. On a trip to Stonehenge, for example, we may ask questions like: How far away is Stonehenge? How long will it take? These questions focus on the goal or the act of reaching the goal. Far less time is spent exploring the nature and meaning of a desire to visit.

Just as on a journey, the language of SFBT presupposes success,[10] in that once the goal is agreed as realistic and achievable (through being curious about a person's past experience of success, the resources that are available to them, their motivation and their confidence), the practitioner uses questions that suggest the goal will be achieved.

A solution focused conversation starts with non-problem talk, the purpose being to establish a relationship with the person and acknowledge that they have a degree of competence in dealing with life outside the problem. The practitioner's side of the conversation consists of asking questions, listening actively and attentively to the answer and building the next question from the given response. The answers to questions asked may reveal clues to, and ultimately create and reveal, solutions.

The practitioner makes no judgements about what the right answer is to the questions that are asked, and takes a 'not-knowing' position. It is argued[11] that since solutions emerge from the person's own expert knowledge of themselves, and are constructed by the question-and-answer conversation, the relationship is one of a 'curious' practitioner and an 'expert' individual. The tone of a solution focused conversation is one of collaboration and acceptance of the person's experience and expertise about the situation.

Case study 10.1: Part I

Vic is a solution focused practitioner, working alongside Rob. In this transcript (Table 10.1), questions are constructed in response to answers given, and the solution focused approach influences what is being asked. Vic and Rob have already engaged in some non-problem talk and have started to chat about the reasons they are meeting.

TABLE 10.1 Solution focuses talk and responses

Session transcript	Commentary
Rob: My CPN [community psychiatric nurse] thought it would be a good idea if I came to see you. She's on my back because I ended up in hospital again.	
Vic: So you're sort of a regular then?	
Rob: Yes . . . embarrassing really, but things get on top of me.	
Vic: How do you cope?	This is a **coping question** that asks Rob how he manages the difficulty. It is intended to help him to recognise existing strategies. Vic does not seek more information about the things that 'get on top of' Rob.
Rob: By drinking . . . a lot. They say I've got to stop but it's really hard – never really done anything else.	

(continued)

Session transcript	Commentary
Vic: So what needs to happen so that you can stop?	This is a straightforward question that is directly eliciting a solution. Vic adopts a 'not-knowing' stance. The assumption is that Rob may know how to stop, or will say if it's too difficult a solution.
Rob: (laughs) If I knew that I would stop, wouldn't I?	
Vic: (laughs) Yes, I guess so . . . although no harm in thinking about it for a while.	The early part of this conversation has created discussion about not drinking. Vic continues to explore whether it is Rob's goal.
Rob: I think about it all the time but I don't get anywhere.	
Vic: You do? You think about it all the time? You must really want to stop drinking?	This is reinforcing Rob's desire to change.
Rob: I do, it's just that it all gets too much for me and it's too easy for me to buy.	Rob reminds Vic that it's too early to establish *not drinking* as his goal.

Case study 10.2: Part II

Vic continues to set a collaborative tone and assists Rob to establish and clarify his goal (Table 10.2). No potential leads towards a solution are dismissed or ignored. Each moves Rob a little closer to expressing a realistic and achievable reason to begin to change. This extract also sees Rob beginning to identify 'What helps' (existing strengths and strategies), and beginning to think about how he copes with difficulties.

TABLE 10.2 What helps and coping

Session transcript	Commentary
Vic: So let me ask you a question. What would need to happen so that the CPN would get off your back?	Vic recalls that Rob identified an early **goal** of keeping the CPN 'off his back'. This is accepted as a reasonable goal. It is used to engage Rob in a conversation on 'what needs to happen'.
Rob: Well she won't ever really, will she? They've got me on those risperidone injections, and I have to take them or the voices get really bad.	

(continued)

Session transcript	Commentary
Vic: So choosing to take the injections helps you with the voices?	Identifying helpful strategies.
Rob: In some ways . . .	
Vic: Tell me in what ways . . .	Vic seeks a positive response, rather than explore injections as a problem. Positive benefits, already suggested by Rob, are sought.
Rob: The voices don't bother me and are quieter. They start to get loud again the day before the injection and that's when I really feel bad.	
Vic: So the injections help with the voices for most of the week?	Vic reinforces a positive strategy by asking for more detail about it. This is also a **coping question**.
Rob: Yeah but it's not enough, and don't ask me to take more medication.	
Vic: OK . . . How do you manage when it starts to get bad again?	This is another **coping question**, seeking to elicit additional helpful strategies and solutions that do not rely on medication.
Rob: Sometimes I take to my bed and try and sleep but that doesn't always help; sometimes I go out, but people look at me – sometimes I tell them to f**k off. Nothing works really.	
Vic: But you keep trying?	Vic says this with approving surprise. Implying that despite the difficulty there is a determination in Rob.

The purpose of solution focused questions mean that they have a different form and structure to questions that are designed to assess the problem. Solution therapists call this *solution talk*[10] and play up the distinction between this type of conversation and the problem-oriented talk that usually takes place. Various questions are used during the conversation. Some, such as the 'miracle question', contribute to goal setting and creating a more positive future view, while others elicit ideas of 'coping'; explore the seeds of solutions by exploring 'exceptions'; contextualise the benefit of change by examining 'relationships'; and use 'scales' that help establish and reinforce small signs of change.

GOAL-SETTING QUESTIONS

> ### Case study 10.3: Part III
>
> The practitioner asks questions in a way that encourages change-focused talk rather than problem talk. The focus is on helping the individual to discover what their preferred future is – that is, re-establishing the person's goals, dreams and ambitions (Table 10.3).

TABLE 10.3 Seeking a preferred future

Session transcript	Commentary
Vic: Let me ask you something. It's a funny question but there is a point to it. Imagine that you go to bed tonight and a miracle happens to you . . .	Vic asks the '**miracle question**', in the style that is used by Insoo Kim Berg.[8] The focus is not on a miracle, but the changes that a miracle brings. Some practitioners use a question that focuses on what the individual hopes for, or use the concept of magical transformation (wishes, magic wand and so forth) to encourage people to describe their preferred future. In all cases, and whatever question is asked, the practitioner is helping the individual to identify what would be different if the problem ceased. It is these differences that are most helpful in describing how an individual wants their life to be better – not the miracle itself.
Rob: Ha (laughs)	
Vic: I told you it was a funny question . . . you go to bed and while you are asleep a miracle happens . . .	
The miracle means that when you wake up your life has changed for the better. Tell me, what would be the first thing you notice that would tell you that today was the first day of the rest of your life?	
Rob: . . . That's hard. No one has ever asked me that before . . . It depends I suppose where I fall asleep.	
Vic: That's true. Where are you sleeping tonight?	
Rob: Could be on the sofa; could be in the bed or could be at the park . . . which means I may wake up in A&E [accident and emergency department] – you see?	
Vic: Let's say, just for tonight, it's in your bed. So if you wake up tomorrow in your own bed and this miracle has happened . . . how would you know.	Vic helps Rob to focus on the question and not get sidetracked by another problem.
Rob: I'd be with someone beautiful.	

(continued)

Session transcript	Commentary
Vic: OK! Anyone you know?	
Rob: (laughs) Paris Hilton!	
Vic: Well it's your miracle. Would you like to have someone special in your life?	Vic does not dismiss the impossible! He explores the difference while acknowledging the fantasy.
Rob: I dunno. Not really.	
Vic: OK. So what would it be like when you open your eyes on the morning after this miracle? What would be different?	
Rob: The voices wouldn't be there.	
Vic: That would be a miracle?	
Rob: Yeah, a real miracle.	
Vic. So what would it be like waking up without the voices? What would be different?	
Rob: I would really be on edge.	
Vic: On edge? Is that a miracle?	
Rob: . . . I guess the miracle would be that I don't have the voices and I would be OK.	
Vic: So what would that be like? If you woke up and the voices were gone and you were OK?	Vic persistently seeks positive differences that indicate a **preferred future**, rather than encouraging Rob to focus on problems.
Rob: It's hard to imagine.	
Vic: So what would you do?	Vic encourages more solution talk, rather than facilitate more discussion about hearing voices.
Rob. Well my life would be more like normal people's.	
Vic: So life would be normal . . . what would you do?	Vic concentrates hard on trying to elicit the changes that would have happened after a miracle. Rob begins to talk about how he wants his life to be, rather than how difficult it is to change.
Rob: It would be normal to wake up without hearing the voices and not feeling sick. Perhaps I would get out of bed instead of lying there until the afternoon.	Rob begins to describe concrete changes to his behaviour . . .
Vic: And what would you do after you got out of bed?	. . . and Vic continues to seek more detail.

EXCEPTION AND COPING QUESTIONS

> ### Case study 10.4: Part IV
> These questions are used to help the person rediscover dormant resources, or uncover resources that they are not aware are available to them. These are often about how the person coped and got through great difficulties in the past, or explore exceptions – times when the immediate problem facing the person has less impact on the current daily experience. While providing individuals with an opportunity to rediscover strengths and abilities, they also bring with them a perspective of change and movement that a person is free to accept of their own volition (Table 10.4).

TABLE 10.4 Exception finding and resource building

Session transcript	Commentary
Vic: Tell me, are there any times, no matter how small, when parts of this miracle happen, or times when things feel a little bit better?	Having established a preferred future, Vic explores whether Rob subconsciously knows how to achieve part of it. This is an **exception question**.
Rob: It's worse when the medication gets out of my system; that's when things get bad.	
Vic: So what about the times before that, before it gets out of your system. Are there any days when you walk down the road not swearing and feeling OK with the world?	Vic focuses on times when the established helpful strategy of taking his medication is being applied. The focus remains on solutions rather than problems.
Rob: Yeah . . . I guess so, people know me around the place. The ones that know me know I'm no trouble, so they stop and talk to me . . . like I'm normal sometimes. Sometimes they ask me how I am when I'm not normal.	
Vic: . . . so they stop and talk and treat you like normal . . . how come?	Vic tries to elicit the presence of positive and helpful behaviour that fits with his preferred future.
Rob: I don't know what's in their heads do I.	
Vic: No . . . of course . . . I meant about you, what do they see that makes you OK to talk to in the street. That's rare these days isn't it?	Another **exception**-seeking question.

(continued)

Session transcript	Commentary
Rob: I like to chat to people – I say 'all right' to them and I get a nod back. I log it then. And when I see them again I ask them where they've been – I get on with them. If they don't respond I don't bother them again.	Rob describes how he is able to interact with people. He is reminded of his personal abilities and qualities. Vic's intention has been to help Rob to notice and remember useful strategies.
Vic: So am I right in asking about this stuff – talking to people is like a small part of this miracle?	Vic is confirming that the conversation is helpful that they are talking about the right things.
Rob: Yeah . . .	
Vic: So what else do you do that is like a small part of this miracle?	One exception is never enough; Vic continues to try to elicit further **exceptions** and positives that Rob may be able to use to improve his life.

RELATIONSHIP QUESTIONS

Solution focused therapy is sometimes described as systemic[11] because it is more interested in change within the person's real world, not inside the therapy room. Questions are asked about how other people would observe the differences if changes are made. These help to contextualise solutions in the person's life. For people experiencing mental health–substance use problems, behaviour may be closely associated with their social situation, so an exploration of the changes that will occur within it is particularly significant.

Case study 10.5: Part V

Here there is a more detailed description of the preferred future – using relationship questions and working with Rob's goal (Table 10.5).

TABLE 10.5 Preferred future and goals

Session transcript	Commentary
If I were to bump into you tomorrow, in the street, and this change had happened and you woke up without voices and your life was more like you want it to be . . . what would I see that would make me think you've really transformed yourself . . . made your life better?	Vic helps Rob to imagine an external picture of himself after the problem has gone. The intention is to help Rob visualise the benefits of changing.

(continued)

Session transcript	Commentary
Rob: You wouldn't recognise me, mate. I'd be like beaming. I'd be walking down the street without swearing at the voices and I'd go across to you and say, Oi Oi! Look at me now mate.	
Vic: What would your CPN say?	
Rob: She would be amazed because I would be tidy and sober – she'd have nothing to say cos all she says is how I have to stop drinking, but what she doesn't understand is that the voices don't go away . . .	This is a **relationship question**; Rob's CPN is used because Rob introduced her as someone who needs to see a difference in him. Rob describes himself as having done something to get her 'off his back' to some extent. This establishes the preferred future within Rob's desires.

SCALING QUESTIONS

Case study 10.6: Part VI

Solution focused practitioners also use language to create questions that are designed to suggest movement and change. The person with the problem is asked to place themselves on a scale (from 0 or 1 to 10), which is often used to ascertain where someone is 'now' and/or their levels of motivation and/or confidence (Table 10.6). The intention of the scale is to help the person to recognise that sometimes change is a process of small constructive steps rather than a sudden transformational event.

TABLE 10.6 Using scales

Session transcript	Commentary
Vic: . . . Let me ask you another strange question then. On a scale of one to ten, where 10 is your perfect life after a miracle and 1 is the worst your life has been . . . which is, I suppose, when you get so drunk you fall over . . .	**Scaling questions** are ultimately intended to break down goals into smaller, more achievable steps. The opening question defines the parameters of the scale. But using this scale, Vic misunderstands how serious Rob feels the bottom of it can be.
Rob: No, that's not it.	
Vic: Uh-uh?	
Rob: The worst moment is when they section me for it again and I end up on the ward.	

(continued)

Session transcript	Commentary
Vic: OK. So that's what you want to avoid. That 1 on a scale is when you end up being sectioned again?	Vic accepts what Rob describes as '1' and reinforces the idea of not wanting it to happen. Change is oriented towards the preferred future.
Rob: Yeah. Definitely.	
Vic: OK, so today . . . on that scale . . . where are you now . . . 10 is a perfect life and one is the worst . . .?	
Rob: Dunno. 4 I guess.	
Vic: 4?	
Rob: Yes.	
Vic: So what's good now that means you are on 4 and not 3?	This question is a further **exception question**. Rob's reply that he is on '4' suggests that he is doing something helpful that prevents the worst thing happening.
Rob: Well I'm not sectioned, I'm not in hospital and I can do what I like.	
Vic: So freedom is important?	
Rob: Oh yes.	
Vic: And what else?	
Rob: I haven't had a drink since the injection two days ago	
Vic: So not drinking, and the injection helps you get to 4?	Positive and helpful behaviour is reinforced.
Rob: Yes.	
Vic: And what else?	
Rob: I've been out and about seeing people.	Rob confirms that his earlier description of exceptions actually does help him to avoid admission to hospital.
Vic: Good . . . anything else?	
Rob: No.	
Vic: So are these things that you need to keep doing to stay at 4?	Reinforcement of existing strategies.
Vic: I mean . . . for as long as you can?	
Rob: I guess so.	

(continued)

Session transcript	Commentary
Vic: Does it ever get better than 4? Have there been times when it was higher than that?	Vic is trying to help Rob to identify other helpful strategies.
Rob: Yeah. When I get off section it's brilliant. Like I can see a whole new life ahead of me. Doesn't last though.	
Vic: But it happens . . . how come?	Vic has noticed that Rob has a keen and repeated desire to change. Asking 'how come' is an attempt to reinforce that desire.
Rob: It's like a clean slate. I can start all over. I promise myself I won't drink again and get in that state but I fall off the wagon.	
Vic: You really want things to be different don't you . . . I will come back to that in a minute. What needs to happen, do you think, for you to move more slowly and steadily up that scale; so that you don't dive straight for 10 but gradually make small, solid changes that will get you closer to it?	Vic stays focused on Rob's desire for things to be different. This is noted and reinforced. Vic introduces the idea of introducing small, achievable changes.
Rob: I don't know.	
Vic: Let's see how it may be possible. What would 5 look like? What would you be doing if you were at 5?	
Rob: I think I would get a job . . .	
Vic: Mmmm . . . that sounds more like a ten to me! Is it possible that you could get a job?	Rob has set himself a goal that is a long way from just speaking to people in the street. Vic attempts to scale this down.
Rob: Yeah, maybe you are right. So 5, yeah?	
Vic: Yeah . . . just a small step.	
Rob: Perhaps I wouldn't be in such a rush to get the drink down me.	
Vic: What do you mean? Drink less?	This is a question that seeks to clarify a smaller, more achievable goal.
Rob: I don't know about that . . . maybe. At the moment the first time I get the voices coming back I go and get a drink. Perhaps if I were stronger I wouldn't give in so quickly.	

(*continued*)

Session transcript	Commentary
Vic: So you would be stronger at 5? How would you get stronger?	
Rob: The voices always win. They tell me what to do and I do it. I could stand up to them more.	
Vic: How would you do that?	
Rob: I don't know.	Rob has ideas about what to do, but doesn't know how to achieve it.
Vic: So let me get this clear. You would like to be able to stand up more to the voices, and this would stop you drinking so quickly and that would be 5 on the scale if you could do that?	
Rob: Yes.	
Vic: So what would you be doing if you were stronger?	Vic starts **goal-setting** questions once more. This time focusing Rob on the goal of being stronger. The question techniques and the conversation continue until Rob is comfortable to experiment with trying to achieve one small step towards his goal of living a more 'normal' life, in which he has more freedom, the continuing threat of hospital admission is lessened and his CPN is less intrusive in his life.

In mental health–substance use problems, practitioners often see the solution as simple: stop the addiction or limit the effects of the mental illness and this will allow the person to change. **SFBT** practitioners recognise that change may need to occur before a person can achieve their own goal – maybe a shift in attitude or beliefs, or simply doing something differently.

TASK SETTING: FROM SOLUTION TALK TO MAKING CHANGES

Meetings may end with agreement between the person and the practitioner about future activity. The idea is simple: change requires an active process that happens in the real world, and it is easy to be sidetracked by problems when faced with every-day life. The point of setting a task is to try to help the person to stay focused on creating their solution. A general guide to setting a task is that *doing* something to change is much harder to achieve than *thinking* about changing, or *noticing* small things that are helpful. People with low motivation should not be asked to do things that are too difficult for them to achieve.

CONCLUSION

Traditional problem-solving methodologies are based on cause and effect; they regard solutions as being the polar opposites of diagnosed problems. However, the individual problems of mental health–substance use act on each other synergistically to create a complicated and sometimes intractable situation. With 'complex needs' such as these, approaches focusing only on the diagnosed problems, rather than on the individual's own hopes and desires, risk preventing the individual from taking control over any part of her/his life.

Resolution is highly dependent on dealing effectively with the most difficult tasks; that is, removing the problems and the associated behaviour, and gaining insight and understanding of the impact of self-destructive behaviour. Anyone who has worked alongside people with such *complicated* problems as these knows that potential failure is ever-present.

Solution focused approaches break with traditional methods and solution focused practitioners construct a different view of the person. The behaviours associated with the problem are seen as unhelpful solution attempts. Practitioners try to help the person to harness and control change, so that it goes in the direction of their goals. Through a series of questioning conversations, the person is helped to learn about their abilities, strengths and resources despite their problems, and then encouraged to make one small step towards their preferred future. Multiple problems, no matter how complex, do not have to prevent a person taking control and making changes in all parts of their life. By staying focused on helping the person to recognise helpful activity, solution focused practitioners encourage small changes that have the potential to cause ripples on an apparently still pool. By remaining confident that the person is capable of change, talking about hopes, noticing and paying attention to resilience and refusing to become enmeshed in the person's problems, change becomes more than a possibility.

REFERENCES

1 Rethink/Turning Point. *Dual Diagnosis Toolkit: mental health and substance misuse.* London: Turning Point; 2004. Available at: www.rethink.org/dualdiagnosis/pdfs/Toolkit. pdf (accessed 6 October 2010).

2 Berg I. In: Popescu B. Paradigm shift in the therapeutic approach: an overview of solution-focused brief therapy. *Europe's Journal of Psychology.* 2005; **1**. Available at: www.ejop.org/archives/2005/02/paradigm_shift_1.html (accessed 12 October 2010).

3 Milner J, O'Byrne P. *Brief Counselling: narratives and solutions.* New York: Palgrave; 2002.

4 Murphy JJ. Solution-focused brief therapy in the school. In: Miller SD, Hubble MA, Duncan BL, editors. *Handbook of Solution-Focused Brief Therapy.* San Francisco: Jossey-Bass; 1996.

5 De Shazer S. *Keys to Solutions in Brief Therapy.* London: WW Norton; 1985.

6 Selekman MD. *Pathways to Change: brief therapy solutions with difficult adolescents.* London: Guildford Press; 1993.

7 Sharry J, Darmody M, Madden B. A solution-focused approach to working with clients who are suicidal. *British Journal of Guidance & Counselling.* 2002; **30**: 383–99.

8 Berg IK, Miller SD. *Working with the Problem Drinker: a solution focused approach.* New York, NY: WW Norton; 1992.

9 McFarland B. *Brief Therapy and Eating Disorders: a practical guide to solution-focused work with clients.* San Francisco: Jossey-Bass; 1995.

10 Hawkes D, Marsh TI, Wilgosh R. *Solution Focused Therapy: a handbook for health care professionals.* London: Butterworth Heinemann; 1998.

11 De Shazer S, Dolan Y, Korman H, *et al. More Than Miracles: the state of the art of solution-focused brief therapy.* New York, NY: Haworth Press; 2007.

TO LEARN MORE

- European Brief Therapy Association

  EBTA holds an annual conference and makes research grants available. Their website includes information and links to other organisations within Europe. Available at: www.ebta.nu/ (accessed 24 January 2011).

- United Kingdom Association of Solution Focused Therapy

  The UKASFP is a membership organisation that promotes the use of SFBT, campaigns for research and wider recognition and publishes *Solution News*, a regular bulletin, and the *Solution Focused Research Review*. Networking is encouraged through the annual conference. Available at: www.ukasfp.co.uk (accessed 24 January 2011).

- The Brief Therapy Institute of Sydney

  Contains an excellent resource page, including session checklists and articles on the approach with many client groups, including people on 'detoxification' programmes. Available at: www.brieftherapysydney.com.au/ (accessed 24 January 2011).

- Anglia Ruskin University

  This University, based in Peterborough, Cambridge and Chelmsford, UK, offers an accredited module at degree level. The module has a focus on practical application of the approach in secondary care settings. For more information contact: dave.hawkes@anglia.ac.uk. Workshops and training for workplace teams are also available.

- BRIEF

  Based in London, BRIEF provides training with in-house certification. Courses are available for therapy and counselling, life coaching and applications in education. Available at: www.brief.org.uk (accessed 24 January 2011).

- Solution Focused Approaches

  The website of Dr Alasdair Macdonald. He provides an SFBT evaluation list, outlining the best of current research into the approach. Available at: www.solutionsdoc.co.uk/ (accessed 24 January 2011).

- More Than Miracles

  Published shortly before Steve de Shazer's death, this book provides a thorough overview of the developments of the approach over 20+ years. It is an excellent resource for the beginner and the more experienced solution focused practitioner: de Shazer S, Dolan Y, Korman H, *et al. More Than Miracles: the state of the art in solution-focused brief therapy.* Abingdon: Routledge; 2007.

CHAPTER 11

Integrated motivational interviewing and cognitive behavioural intervention

Michael Fitzsimmons and Christine Barrowclough

INTRODUCTION

KEY POINT 11.1

The combination of psychosis and substance use problems is common.

Substance use in people with schizophrenia is common. Estimates of lifetime prevalence of drug use, harmful alcohol drinking or substance dependence (substance use) for individuals with schizophrenia are around 50%.[1,2] Poor clinical and social outcomes, failure to access treatment or inadequate treatment delivery is not uncommon.[3-7] Drug and alcohol problems have been shown to be among the most important predictors for frequent rehospitalisation.[8-10] Increased rates of aggression and violence,[11,12] increased risk of death by suicide[13,14] and an increased risk of social exclusion are all associated with psychosis–substance use problems.

Engagement in treatment is often difficult and studies indicate that attrition rates are high, even for those agreeing to come into treatment.[15,16] Contributory factors may include a bias towards suspiciousness or paranoid interpretation of relationships arising from the psychotic symptoms and exacerbated by substance use, and a chaotic lifestyle along with concurrent problems make appointment scheduling and engaging in structured work more difficult.[17]

Because of the negative impact of substance use on psychosis, in recent years there has been much interest in trying to understand what the most effective approaches are to working with these individuals. The consensus is that integrated treatment should be the standard approach for evidence-based treatment.[18]

> **KEY POINT 11.2**
>
> Integrated treatment approaches drawn from both substance use and mental health fields are recommended.

Integrated treatment describes a flexible combination of treatments from the mental health and substance use fields that are blended together in the treatment of an individual experiencing psychosis-substance use disorders. The components of integrated programmes have included motivational interventions, assertive outreach, intensive case management, group and individual counselling and family interventions.[19] However, as previously noted, engagement in treatment is often not the priority for the individual. A common factor contributing to the refusal or avoidance of engagement with treatment is low motivation to reduce substance use.[20,21] While there is growing evidence that substance use may impact negatively on the course of psychosis, the individual may not consider the negative consequences of substance use to outweigh their perceived positive expectancies of continued use. This suggests that interventions need to be flexible to work with individuals at whatever stage they are at in the change process.[22]

There are some indications that motivational interviewing (MI – *see* Book 4, Chapters 6 and 7) can be successfully used with people experiencing psychosis-substance use problems[23] while cognitive behavioural therapy (CBT – *see* Book 4, Chapter 10) has been shown in recent years to be effective[24] for the symptoms of psychosis. The approach developed in Manchester, UK,[21,25] for people experiencing schizophrenia and coexisting drug or alcohol problems (substance use) found better outcomes for a treatment that combined three intervention components – MI, CBT and a family intervention – over a nine-month period, when compared with standard mental healthcare. The interventions from this study have been further developed and are currently being evaluated in a larger randomised controlled trial in the UK – the MIDAS trial.[26]

The focus of this chapter is on the MIDAS therapy approach for psychosis-substance use problems (MiCBT). The approach has already been described in earlier texts;[17,22] this chapter aims to expand on previous descriptions, and provides more detail with an extended case study. The chapter describes the model that underpins the therapeutic approach and reviews the current understanding of interactions between psychosis and substances. The MiCBT approach, which integrates MI with recognised CBT for psychosis, is illustrated through a case study describing the process of integrated therapy for psychosis-substance use problems.

INTERACTIONS BETWEEN PSYCHOSIS AND SUBSTANCE USE

The pattern of substance use in psychosis is similar to that in the general population; namely, alcohol and cannabis are the most commonly used substances and polysubstance use is common.[27] Having a vulnerability to psychosis increases the risk of experiencing negative effects from certain substances[28,29] with adverse negative consequences resulting from lower levels of use than in the general population.[30]

KEY POINT 11.3

People with a diagnosis of psychosis seem to be more vulnerable to the negative effects of substances than those without psychosis.

Substance use by people vulnerable to psychosis can affect them negatively in a number of ways. We have found it useful to separate the negative consequences into either **internal** or **external difficulties**.

➤ **Internal difficulties** include unpleasant withdrawal symptoms, depressed mood, increased perceptual and cognitive anomalies.

➤ **External difficulties** include, for example, interpersonal conflicts associated with the substance use (e.g. with relatives, partners and professionals who disapprove of substance use and blame the individual for worsening his/her situation), or financial and accommodation issues arising from substance use.

The stress associated with these difficulties is likely to further exacerbate psychotic symptoms.[31]

Given the associated complications of psychosis-substance use, why are there high rates of substance use among people with schizophrenia? Gregg and colleagues[32] looked at four generally held explanations for the high rates of substance use among people with schizophrenia:

1 substance use causes psychosis.
2 psychosis causes substance use.
3 substance use and psychosis share a common origin.
4 psychosis and substance use interact and maintain each other.

They concluded that there are probably multiple risk factors involved in substance use in psychosis and that although these four general explanations may have previously helped to clarify the understanding of the reasons for substance use by people with schizophrenia, no single model is able to adequately explain all comorbidity. Different models may account for comorbidity in different groups of people while multiple models may apply for other individuals. The social context and accessibility of substances is what most often dictates the choice of substance in psychosis[33,34] rather than selection of a particular substance to relieve particular symptoms of psychosis – that is, the self-medication theory.[35] Nonetheless, self-reports indicate that situations and cues triggering use may be related to some of the negative consequences of the disorder, particularly dysphoria and distress, or to symptoms such as paranoia or hearing voices.[3,36]

Reasons given for use of substances by people with psychosis do not differ from those of the general population;[37] for example:

➤ being accepted by a social group
➤ personal choice
➤ wanting something different out of life
➤ response to negative affective states

➤ interpersonal conflict
➤ social pressures.[38,39]

Gregg and colleagues[36] identified three distinct reasons for substance use among people with a diagnosis of schizophrenia:
1 for social and enhancement reasons, to 'chill out and have a good time with others'
2 to regulate negative affect and alleviate positive symptoms, and to 'cope with distressing emotions and symptoms'
3 to intensify their experiences, to 'feel bigger, better and inspired.'

A HEURISTIC MODEL OF PSYCHOSIS AND SUBSTANCE USE

An integrated model of the relationships between psychosis and substance use is helpful to inform the process of MiCBT and to provide a framework for understanding the potential links between psychosis and repeated substance use. The model developed for use in the MIDAS approach (Figure 11.1) incorporates Marlatt and Gordon's[38] social-cognitive theory of problematic substance use, with elements of Blanchard and colleagues'[3] model of the relationship between substance use and psychosis, as well as recent research concerning the links between psychosis and drug or alcohol problems.

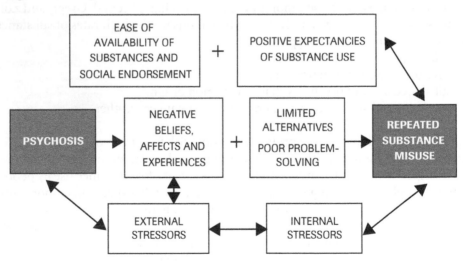

FIGURE 11.1 MIDAS model of maintenance of substance use in schizophrenia

Psychosis brings with it a number of associated difficulties:
➤ increased intensity and distress from voice hearing
➤ increased levels of anxiety
➤ increased levels of paranoid thinking
➤ difficulties with concentration
➤ increased risk of conflict with family members
➤ unwanted admissions to hospital.

In this context, poor problem-solving abilities[40] and limited ways of obtaining pleasure other than through substance use, tend to reinforce expectation of the positive benefits of repeated substance use. We have found in clinical practice that the contributing role of substance use to associated psychosis difficulties may not be as significant to the individual as to other concerned people – that is, family, mental health services, criminal justice system. Rather, substance use is more likely to be associated with positive than negative expectancies, leading to a situation in which substance use is maintained.

In a qualitative study of reasons for substance use in a sample of individuals with recent onset psychosis, Lobbana and colleagues[41] identified a number of reasons why substance use is maintained:

➤ an increased availability of substances once a particular social network was established around drug use
➤ a perception of shared experience and membership that is reinforced as relationships and networks grow around drug-using communities
➤ an increased sense of detachment from non-drug-using networks and related fear of isolation should existing group membership be severed.

Other perceived positive expectancies of continued substance use may include opportunity to reduce boredom, reducing levels of anxiety, blocking out distressing thoughts and helping with sleep difficulties.[17]

The heuristic model described here is used to guide the therapeutic approach (MiCBT) described later in this chapter. Using the model as a template helps the therapist to complete a detailed functional analysis of the links between the person's psychosis-associated difficulties and their continued substance use, by eliciting this information at distinct stages of the therapeutic intervention (*see* Book 4, Chapter 2). The model helps the therapist to elicit self-motivational statements from the individual regarding the negative aspects of continued substance use and to then feed this back through a shared understanding.

TREATMENT APPROACHES
Motivational challenges and approaches
Designing effective treatment strategies targeting psychosis-substance use disorders presents considerable challenges.[42] It is not unusual for individuals to be ambivalent about:

➤ engagement with services
➤ adherence to treatment
➤ their mental health diagnosis
➤ reducing substance use.

This ambivalence is often seen by services as evidence that the individual is either unmotivated to change or is lacking in insight, which further compounds the difficulties of engagement in treatment as this approach is likely to create resistance from the individual.

> **KEY POINT 11.4**
>
> Ambivalence about engaging in therapeutic approaches is common.

There has been particular emphasis on applying motivational interventions – and in particular motivational interviewing (MI) – to take account of the individual's motivation to address or reduce their substance use and to engage in the therapeutic process.[18,43,44] It is not the intention of this chapter to provide a comprehensive description of MI, there being a number of texts and resources to which the reader can refer (*see* Book 4, Chapters 6 and 7).[43,45] Nonetheless, it will be useful to provide a brief description of the approach.

Miller and Rollnick define MI as 'a client-centred, directive method for enhancing intrinsic motivation to change by exploring and resolving ambivalence'.[43] Motivational interviewing was originally conceptualised as a therapeutic approach to guide people from precontemplation or contemplation into preparation and action, by increasing motivation and commitment to change.[46] In the MI approach, the individual is generally viewed as feeling highly ambivalent about changing. Building intrinsic motivation for change involves the therapist selectively eliciting and reinforcing 'change talk'.[47] Change talk is the individual's own arguments and motivations for *change* as opposed to 'sustain talk', which is the individual's own arguments and motivations for *no change*.

Rollnick and colleagues[48] identify six categories of change talk: DARN–CT.
1 **Desire** – statements about preference for change.
2 **Ability** – statements about capability of change.
3 **Reasons** – specific arguments for change.
4 **Need** – statements about feeling obliged to change.
5 **Commitment** – statements about the likelihood of change.
6 **Taking steps** – statements about action being taken.

> **KEY POINT 11.5**
>
> Approaches need to be flexible to take account of ambivalence to participate in treatment, and low motivation to reduce substance use.

The therapist using a motivational interviewing approach will selectively elicit and reinforce change talk through the use of core MI skills – OARS:
➤ **O**pen questions
➤ **A**ffirmations
➤ **R**eflective listening
➤ **S**ummary.

Motivational interviewing aims to build motivation to change through the use of four principles:

1   rolling with resistance
2   developing discrepancy
3   expressing empathy
4   supporting self-efficacy.

The therapy is delivered within a framework of Autonomy, Collaboration, and Evocation, referred to as MI spirit, which has the following features:
➤   **Autonomy** – the therapist affirms the individual's right and capacity for self-direction and facilitates informed choice.
➤   **Collaboration** – a partnership is delivered that honours the individual's expertise and perspectives.
➤   **Evocation** – recognises that the resources and motivation for change lie within the individual.

Adapting motivational interviewing for psychosis

MI seems well suited for people experiencing psychosis-substance use disorders because of the primary importance of engagement and motivational strategies.[49–53] Some modification of MI practice is necessary to address the complex needs of those experiencing psychosis-substance use disorders. Barrowclough and colleagues[17] recommend:
➤   using less complex reflections
➤   detouring emotional material that may lead to distressing 'psychotic' symptoms
➤   providing sufficient time for the individual to respond to reflections and summaries
➤   making more use of frequent and short reflections to clarify meaning
➤   avoiding complicated language and multiple choices by using simple, open questions.

Martino and Moyers[54] further suggest that written specific activities may be necessary to structure the sessions, such as using balance sheets to explore the good things and not-so-good things about substances, and ruler scales to elicit confidence and the importance of change.

It may be that individuals have been told on many occasions that their substance use is compromising their treatment and that they need to abstain or at the very least reduce their use of substances. This can lead to the individual feeling 'nagged at', resulting in a tendency to say what other people want to hear. From clinical experience, we have found that it is important to take a conservative approach to moving forward with change[22] to consolidate the individual's own intrinsic motivation to change and to identify barriers to change.

Integrating motivational interviewing with cognitive behavioural therapy

The MIDAS therapy approach described in more detail later in this chapter integrates MI and recognised CBT for psychosis approaches.[24,55,56] CBT as an approach for people with psychosis has been shown to be helpful in re-evaluating perceptions, beliefs, thinking styles and unhelpful behaviours related to distressing psychotic experiences and associated emotional difficulties, and as such is recommended as an appropriate treatment option.[57] The benefit of integrating MI and CBT is in ensuring that all elements of the problems are given attention and any negative interactions between mental health and substance use problems can be formulated and addressed while taking into account the person's motivation to address or reduce their substance use.

Integrating MI and CBT is not unique to the MIDAS approach. While (for substance use and psychosis) it has been more common to use them sequentially (first MI as a pre-treatment phase, then CBT) in recent years a number of authors[44,54,58] have described the use of MI in conjunction with CBT for a number of disorders, using an integrative framework. Motivational interviewing and CBT share similar approaches to working with clinical problems; both are rooted in the Socratic method of eliciting rather than imposing information, and both are person-centred and emphasise the need to respect autonomy. A significant difference is that CBT interventions often assume from the outset that the person is motivated to change and do not explicitly address issues relating to ambivalence within therapy, or have techniques available to do so. Difficulties associated with low motivation and resistance can appear at any point in therapy. Having the flexibility to switch to a more MI style may help to resolve any resistance, increase motivation and, in turn, contribute to more positive engagement and better outcomes.[59]

MICBT: THE MIDAS THERAPY APPROACH

The MIDAS therapy approach is built around two therapy phases. Phase one is concerned with building motivation to change and developing a shared understanding of how the person's life concerns fit with psychosis-substance use problems. Once the individual has made a commitment to change, phase two then focuses on developing a plan that can be implemented to reduce substance use, and to identify more effective ways of managing high-risk situations or symptoms that may lead to relapse. It is expected that in phase one there will be more use of MI strategies to build and consolidate motivation to change, whereas in phase two there will be much more of an emphasis on CBT approaches to address high-risk situations for relapse, particularly difficulties associated with psychosis.

Both phases have a number of stages described later in this chapter. While it is expected that the therapist and individual attempt to work through each stage, there is likely to be variation dependent upon individual circumstances and the stage of change the person is at regarding engagement in therapy and motivation to reduce substance use. For the person who is ready to reduce substance use, it will be more appropriate to move on to phase two after a relatively brief review of phase one stages. On the other hand, as has been more usual in our clinical experience, the individual who is ambivalent about meeting for therapy may require brief but frequent visits to develop engagement before it is possible to work through the phases and begin looking at how their concerns fit into their psychosis and substance use.

1 Building engagement and helping the individual to explore concerns, values and satisfactions

A number of reasons may underlie initial difficulties with engagement. There may be stigma issues and/or psychotic phenomena that limit development of trust. There may be previous negative experiences associated with trusting others and/or unpleasant or unhelpful therapeutic contacts in the past. If motivation to engage in treatment is not seen as a priority, it is crucial that the therapist spends time eliciting the individual's thoughts about being in therapy. This gives the therapist the opportunity to provide information about what therapy may entail, and to assess the individual's motivation to be in therapy.

SELF-ASSESSMENT EXERCISE 11.1

Time: 5 minutes
Think about the type of questions you will need to ask.

Examples of questions that could be asked are:
➤ What are your thoughts about being here today?
➤ What concerns do you have about meeting with me?
➤ What would you like to get out of our meetings?
➤ Would it be OK if I told you what the meeting may involve?

If the person repeatedly misses appointments, the therapist should explore their reasons for this. Non-attendance may be a consequence of ambivalent feelings about therapy. It is important to keep in mind that, even if the person agreed to therapy, people do change their mind and ambivalence is a normal reaction.

Identifying **goals** and **key values** is not only essential in understanding the person's perspective but also a key component of the engagement process. Strategically, developing intrinsic motivation to change occurs when there is discrepancy between current behaviour and cherished values and goals. Potential examples of discrepancy between values, goals and substance use could be:
➤ the person with a young child who experiences discrepancy between the amount of money they spend on cannabis use and their value of 'contributing financially for my children', especially if money is scarce within the family
➤ the person who values 'socialising' and who identifies that they do not feel able to do so when 'stoned'
➤ the person who values keeping well and staying out of hospital and who also identifies that continued amphetamine use may be problematic to their mental health.

It may be that simply asking 'What are your goals?' or 'What is important to you?' will not result in the individual succinctly identifying a list of cherished values and goals. The therapist will need to carefully elicit and clarify through evocative questioning what are the individual's values and goals. Using the values sort card[60] can also help to elicit what the individual considers to be important in their life.

SELF-ASSESSMENT EXERCISE 11.2

> **Time: 5 minutes**
> Think what questions you might need to ask in order to help elicit key goals and values.

Examples of possible questions that could be asked are:
➤ What do you most enjoy doing with your time?
➤ What do you do during the day that you do not really like doing?
➤ How would you like things to be different?
➤ What things might improve the quality of your life?
➤ How do you see yourself in: 6 months, 12 months, 5 years?

2 Eliciting how substance use fits into concerns, values and life satisfactions

Once the therapist has begun to develop engagement, the aim is then to assist the individual in making links between their substance use and key concerns. It is important that the therapist listens for change statements and reinforces them by the use of selective reflections and summaries. The therapist's style at this stage is to provide a neutral response to any dilemma that the person may be describing. This allows the individual to explore their ambivalence in a non-judgemental relationship. If the person does not think there are any difficulties regarding their substance use, that is fine, as it helps the therapist to assess motivation to change. Clearly if the individual does not see any difficulties, it is unlikely that they are going to be making any changes in the immediate future. Information offered at this stage assists the therapist to elicit the person's stage of change and helps to inform the focus for the rest of the intervention.

3 Eliciting how psychosis fits into this picture

It is important to elicit the individual's understanding of their current situation with respect to onset, symptoms experienced, consequences of psychosis and their understanding of any interactions between their psychosis and their substance use. This needs to take place within a therapeutic alliance in which psychosis and substance use can be discussed openly. It is the aim of the therapist at this stage to elicit from the person any negative associations they themselves have already identified, and to strengthen the individual's awareness of these possible connections and so increase motivation to reduce substance use.

A statement from the individual such as:

> 'Having a smoke in the morning stops me getting wound up by paranoid thoughts, but doesn't make them go away and sometimes actually makes me feel worse'

. . . could be reflected back by the therapist as:

'You really want to stop feeling paranoid and you have some concerns that smoking weed could actually be making things worse in the long term.'

This reflection from the therapist draws on the person's own concerns and understanding. This could then be augmented by giving the person (with permission) some information to help them examine how substance use may fit into their concerns regarding mental health.

Information can be provided in a number of ways, such as:
➤ 'expert' opinion
➤ discussion of pamphlets/booklets/DVDs from personal experiences of people experiencing psychosis-substance use problems
➤ information from specific websites
➤ completing a diary of symptoms in relation to substance use.

4 Sharing of initial understanding/formulation of how life concerns fit together with psychosis and substance use

While the early stages of therapy mainly use MI techniques, sharing an understanding of how things fit together in the person's life requires more integration of MI and CBT. The shared understanding is essentially a cognitive behavioural formulation, and hence it may be appropriate to use CBT techniques to elicit thoughts, feelings and behaviours associated with the onset and maintenance of the problem. The spirit of MI remains throughout, respecting the individual's autonomy and expertise. OARS are used to regularly elicit feedback from the individual and the therapist continues to monitor and respond to resistance.

For all formulations, it will be helpful to use recent examples of difficulties and to describe these in detail, with a focus on:
➤ relevant events
➤ thoughts
➤ feelings
➤ coping
➤ consequences/outcomes.

Levels of complexity of formulations will inevitably vary. For people who do not see substance use as problematic (and for whom it has therefore been inappropriate to gather assessment information about use), there may be only limited understanding of any associations between the substance use and psychosis or other life concerns. On the other hand, therapists need to take great care in considering the degree of complexity individuals will find useful and in tailoring the formulation to meet the individual's needs. A number of factors will determine the complexity of the formulation, such as:
➤ the degree to which the individual has engaged in the shared process of exploration
➤ the amount of information generated/shared between therapist and individual (some will have provided a lot of detail about their concerns, others will have provided very little)

➤ the individual's stage of change in relation to the target change behaviour and the individual's willingness to discuss particular issues
➤ individual differences among people in their ability or desire to describe their experiences.

As a result, the depth or level of formulation will vary widely. However, whatever the complexity, it is usually possible to achieve some sort of shared formulation regardless of the stage in therapy.[61]

MOVING INTO ACTION PHASE

5 Discussion of possible change options

When the therapist and individual have worked on the shared understanding together, key open questions and reflections can be used in order to help explore the information. For example:
➤ Given what you've told me, what do you think you will do next?
➤ Where do you think you would like to go from here?
➤ What's your next step?

The aim at this stage is for the therapist to discuss with the individual their readiness to make a change in their substance use. This discussion will be based upon the information presented in the formulation. At this stage, the therapist is looking to elicit statements of commitment to change. It may be that the individual will be expressing statements of **D**esire, **A**bility, **R**easons or **N**eed (DARN) to change but not expressing *commitment* to change. This suggests that the therapist needs to spend more time eliciting commitment to change. If, however, the individual decides that they are going to make a change in their substance use, then, together with the therapist, the formulation will be reviewed and a change plan developed.

6 Reviewing the formulation and developing a change plan

Once the person decides on the change that they would like to make it is recommended that a written change plan,[43] developed from a revised formulation specifically looking at agreed goals and strategies, is collaboratively agreed upon. The details of the change plan are summarised here.

The change plan
➤ The changes I want to make or continue making are:
➤ The reasons I want to make these changes are:
➤ The steps I plan to take in changing are:
➤ The ways other people can help me are:
➤ I will know my plan is working if:
➤ Some things that could get in the way of my plan are:
➤ What I will do if my plan is not working:

The therapist needs to be aware that ambivalence can reappear at any time; hence, it is essential that the change plan is developed and shared in a truly collaborative way to avoid the individual perceiving the change as external in source rather than intrinsic to them. Strategically, the change plan aims to consolidate motivation to change substance use based on the negative consequences of psychosis-substance use disorders identified in the formulation.

ACTION PHASE
7 CBT intervention identified from formulation

Based on the revised formulation and the change plan a CBT intervention for psychosis-substance use problems will likely include some of the following components:

➤ identifying and increasing awareness of high-risk situations/warning signs that might make lapse/relapse more likely to occur

➤ developing new coping skills for handling such high-risk situations/warning signs, with particular attention to symptom- and mental-health related problems highlighted in the formulation (e.g. strategies for dealing with distressing voices or with depressed mood)

➤ coping with cravings and urges (*see* Book 4, Chapter 13)

➤ making lifestyle changes so as to decrease need/urges for drugs and/or alcohol or to increase healthy activities/alternative options to substance use (e.g. activity planning where boredom or lack of social contact have been identified as key issues, avoiding or limiting contact with substance-using friends and planning alternatives)

➤ normalising lapses and preparing responses to lapses so that they do not result in full-blown relapse

➤ developing strategies and plans for acting in the event of lapse/relapse so that adverse consequences may be minimised

➤ cognitive restructuring around alcohol and drug expectations.

CASE STUDY

The remainder of the chapter will focus on a case study drawn from the authors' clinical experience. The description of the individual, while fairly typical, is disguised so that anonymity is maintained. The case study will attempt to illustrate the process of working through the two phases of therapy, focusing on the different stages of the two phases.

Case study 11.1: Kevin

Kevin (26) has a five-year history of involvement with mental health services. He has a diagnosis of schizophrenia and had been a polysubstance user from the age of 14. Kevin currently uses cannabis daily and alcohol 2–3 times per week dependent upon finances. Kevin tends to use cannabis by himself except when with two friends he met while in hospital who visit a couple of times a week to stay over and have a smoke.

Kevin is the youngest of three children. His father has a history of treatment for bipolar disorder and also alcohol dependency. His relationship with his mother has been inconsistent as she left the family home when Kevin and his two older sisters were young. He is in regular contact with his elder sister. However, she is unhappy about his cannabis use and refuses to let Kevin visit her home due to his use of drugs. Kevin has little contact with anybody else other than the two friends he met while in hospital.

Kevin does not like taking medication and is not wholly convinced that his use of cannabis causes him any difficulties. Kevin has had three hospital admissions all under the UK Mental Health Act. When in hospital he has limited access to cannabis and recovers relatively quickly. Prior to his first episode of psychosis Kevin had been arrested for causing a disturbance at a benefits agency office due to his benefit claim being wrongly processed. Since this time, Kevin has had intrusive paranoid thoughts that he is under surveillance from the benefits agency. Because of these concerns, Kevin avoids going out by himself, isolates himself and fills his time smoking cannabis. He suggests that he smokes cannabis to fill his time because it makes him remember how he used to feel before he became unwell, and to help him generally relax and feel better.

Kevin was initially quite reluctant to engage in therapy as he was unsure how it would help his situation.

Phase one: building motivation to change

The therapist agreed to hold the sessions with Kevin at his flat. From the outset, Kevin stated that he did not want to meet on a regular basis, suggesting that it would be best to meet every 4–6 weeks rather than weekly to fortnightly as suggested by the therapist. The therapist explored this ambivalence about meeting regularly to elicit Kevin's concerns about being involved in therapy.

Therapist – 'You seem to have some doubts about meeting with me. I wonder what they might be.'

Kevin – 'I don't know really . . . I'm not really sure that it will do me any good just talking.'

Therapist – 'Your time is important to you. If you are going to do something it has to be worth your while.'

Kevin – 'All I want is to stay out of hospital. How is just talking about drugs and things going to help?'

Therapist – 'Many people who start therapy are unsure how it might benefit them. If you like I could tell you how other people have used their time in therapy. We could also look at what you think would be a good use of your time. It really is your choice.'

Kevin – 'How has it helped other people?'

Therapist – 'Other people I have worked with have used therapy as an opportunity to identify how they would like their life to be different, and then together we have looked at what might have to change to make it happen.'

Kevin – 'You mean like staying out of hospital?'

Therapist – 'If staying out of hospital is what the person sees as being important to them then we would try to work out together what is getting in the way of them staying out of hospital. What do you think about using our time together in that way?'

Kevin agreed to meet more frequently, being assured that he would be able to decide the length of the sessions. The therapist made a number of fairly short visits to begin with, spending time eliciting Kevin's interests (such as fishing, computer games, listening to music) while also gently encouraging him to talk about his concerns. Staying out of hospital was important to Kevin, as was feeling less paranoid, having more enjoyment from life, and possibly getting a job and then maybe a girlfriend.

Kevin brought up his cannabis use when discussing his ambivalence about therapy.

Kevin – 'So do you just want to bang on about how smoking weed got me into this situation?'

Therapist – 'It seems as though you don't find it helpful when people tell you what to do.'

Kevin – 'Yeah, so how is this going to be any different?'

Therapist – 'My goal for now is just to try and understand what you think is going on in your life. It's clear from our conversations so far that you have a good understanding of what is going on in your life at the moment. Being told by other people that smoking weed has brought about your current difficulties makes you annoyed.'

Kevin – 'It's part of their job to tell you that smoking weed is bad for you. They have to do it.'

Therapist – 'So you are wondering how this is going to be any different.'

Kevin – 'Well, yeah I suppose so.'

Therapist – 'There is some evidence that smoking weed can be unhelpful for some people who have had a psychotic episode, which may be why you are being told this. If you would like, we can talk about that some more. For now though I'm really just interested in knowing a little more about how you think your cannabis use fits into your life.'

Strategically the therapist rolled with Kevin's resistance to gain permission to look at his thoughts about psychosis and substance use in later sessions. In the third session, the therapist picked up on this again.

Therapist – 'You talked about how other people seem to think that smoking cannabis isn't a good idea for you.'

Kevin – 'Why do you think that it isn't good for me?'

Therapist – 'Other people have suggested to you that smoking weed isn't helpful.'

Kevin – 'Yeah, the doctor that comes out to see me says that I'll relapse if I carry on smoking.'

Therapist – 'That worries you.'

Kevin – 'Well it scares me a bit 'cause I don't want to end up in hospital again and there have been a few times recently when I've ended up feeling more paranoid after I've had a smoke, and my sister definitely thinks it is making my paranoia worse. But having a smoke sort of helps me to chill out, and when you have nothing to do it helps the day pass quicker.'

Therapist – 'You are in two minds about whether cannabis is really that bad. The message you have received is that it might not be that helpful but you find that it helps you to chill out. You've mentioned that when you spend time with your friends it seems a good idea to have a smoke to chill out and relax and that when you are bored at home you find that you have a smoke to help pass the time. Other people though seem to think that it is making your psychosis worse, and there have been a few times recently when you have experienced pretty bad paranoia after you have had a smoke.'

Kevin – 'Yeah that's pretty much what's going on.'

Therapist – 'Other people in a similar situation to you have found it useful to focus in a bit more detail on identifying what are the good things and not-so-good things about having a smoke, before they even think about making any decisions. What are your thoughts about trying that out?'

The therapist made it clear that it was the individual's *perspective* that was being sought and not commitment to make a change. Kevin and the therapist then explored his ambivalence through the use of a decision balance analysis (Table 11.1).

TABLE 11.1 Decision balance analysis looking at reducing cannabis use

MAKING A CHANGE	**GOOD THINGS (A)**	**NOT-SO-GOOD THINGS (B)**
	Stop feeling so paranoid	Will not see friends as much
	More money	Might affect my sleep
	Better concentration	Will get bored as I've got nothing else to do with my time
	Take my driving licence and get a car	
		Smoking makes me more alert for danger and if I stop I might end up dropping my guard
	Not having to be dependent on anything to make me feel better	
		I'll miss feeling stoned
	Will get my sisters off my back	
		I'm scared that I'll end up getting angry with people and getting into fights
	Feel as though I've achieved something	
NOT MAKING A CHANGE	**GOOD THINGS (C)**	**NOT-SO-GOOD THINGS (D)**
	It's part of who I am and I don't really like change	The good things are starting to outweigh the bad things
	Still get to see friends	I get a weird buzz these days when I smoke
	I won't have to explain to friends why I'm not having a smoke	
		It will be difficult to smoke and keep a job down
		I'll probably end up back in hospital
		Being stopped by the police
		It affects my concentration

The therapist, while eliciting reasons *not to change* ('sustain talk' – B and C), focused on the reasons *for change* ('change talk' – A and D) to elicit further change talk (Table 11.1). Kevin was asked if it was OK to look in more detail at times when he felt more paranoid and where his cannabis use fitted into those times. A simple diary was proposed in which Kevin recorded the times that he had a smoke and then recorded how he felt during the hour after he had a smoke (Table 11.2).

TABLE 11.2 Diary of use and feelings

Time had a smoke	Mood	Paranoia
e.g. 12:00	0 = worst ever; 10 = best ever	0 = worst ever; 10 = no problems

The following week, although Kevin had only completed his diary on a few occasions he suggested that he had been taking more notice of how his use of cannabis had been making him feel. In session, the therapist attempted to do a retrospective diary of the past few days, which did seem to suggest that Kevin experienced higher levels of anxiety and paranoid thinking following cannabis use. Although the therapist was able to see evidence of some links between increased levels of paranoia and times when using cannabis, Kevin's own conclusions were elicited rather than the therapist pointing out the links.

> Therapist – 'What links do you see between your cannabis use and times when you feel more paranoid?'
> Kevin – 'It looks like if I smoke too much then it does make me more paranoid, which means that I'm making things worse for myself in the long term, but having a smoke is part of who I am.'
> Therapist – 'Continuing to smoke is important to you but it does look like it can make you feel more paranoid.'
> Kevin – 'I suppose if I carry on smoking I'll never be able to get a job. If I'm too paranoid to go out of the house how will I be around people I don't know?'

Over the next two sessions the therapist aimed to look in more detail at Kevin's experience of psychosis – how his cannabis use and other life stressors seemed to adversely affect it day to day – and to collaboratively develop a shared understanding of his current difficulties (Figure 11.2). The shared understanding was developed with Kevin in session. Kevin was invited to fill out the boxes of the model. Although he declined to do this, he remained active in the development of the shared understanding. Kevin identified that feeling paranoid and low in mood were his main difficulties. The therapist elicited that this caused Kevin to think of himself as a failure as he was not in control of his situation, which caused him to feel depressed and scared, and this in turn led to Kevin rarely going out of his flat alone. As a consequence of this, Kevin's paranoia and low mood were maintained. To cope with this Kevin isolated himself further, was hypervigilant to any perceived threats and on occasions became angry with people he believed were 'spying on him', which led to complaints being made by neighbours to the housing department. In this context,

Kevin used cannabis as he expected it to make him feel relaxed, stopped him from getting angry and helped him to remain alert to danger. Cannabis was easy to obtain and his limited social network all used cannabis. However, despite this, Kevin had begun to recognise that using cannabis made him feel anxious and paranoid and he was concerned that it would be detrimental in the long term. Not having a job, the increased risk of being admitted to hospital, spending approximately £600 per month on cannabis, and difficult relationships with his housing providers as well as his sister all contributed to increased stress, which adversely affected his difficulties with paranoia and low mood. Kevin was asked what he made of this formulation (Figure 11.2).

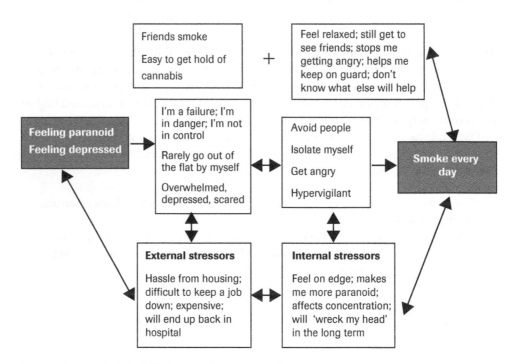

FIGURE 11.2 Kevin's initial shared understanding

Kevin – 'As I said before it all points to having to stop smoking at some point but . . .' [long pause]'
    Therapist – 'You're worried that it might be too difficult.'
    Kevin – 'I know some people who have stopped but I'm not really like them.'
    Therapist – 'In what way?'
    Kevin – 'I've always had difficulty trying to do new things and I can't see how this will be any different.'

Kevin was asked to rate on a scale of '0–10' (Miller and Rollnick,[43] p. 53) how important reducing his cannabis was to him – where '0' = not important at all and '10' = extremely important. Kevin suggested that he was at a '7'. The therapist then asked why he had said '7' and not a lower number such as '2'. Kevin responded with 'change talk'.

> Kevin – 'I want to stay out of hospital; I want to feel less paranoid, think more clearly, improve my memory and have more money to treat myself.'

However, from previous conversations, the therapist had some doubts as to Kevin's own confidence to be able to change. Kevin was asked how confident he was that he could make a significant change in his cannabis use with '0' being not confident at all and '10' being extremely confident. Kevin replied that he was at a '3'. He was then asked why he was at a '3' and not at '0'. The therapist strategically asked Kevin why he did not reply with a lower number, in order to elicit confidence talk – that is, statements reflecting the possibility that change could happen.

> Therapist – 'In terms of how confident you are to make this change, what would you say were the reasons why you put yourself at a '3' and not lower such as '0'?'
> Kevin – 'Well I've been able to stop using amphetamine and I don't drink as much these days as I used to.'
> Therapist – 'This encourages you that you can successfully make changes.'
> Kevin – 'I didn't always smoke as much weed as I do now. I used to be able to control the amount that I smoked.'
> Therapist – 'Looking at your past successes, change seems possible. What else have you succeeded in that gives you confidence?'
> Kevin – 'I've kept my own flat when everyone said I wasn't capable of living by myself.'
> Therapist – 'So looking back you have successfully reduced your alcohol use, stopped using amphetamine, managed to live independently and have previously been able to control the amount of weed you smoke.'

Kevin was then asked what he thought would help him to move from a '3' to a higher number, such as a '6', which again elicited further confidence talk and provided the therapist with a clearer idea of what might help initiate change. Kevin suggested that if he had things to look forward to, something to do with his time, better ways of coping with his paranoid thoughts and a clearer idea of what the risks of reducing cannabis were, his confidence would be increased.

The therapist again asks Kevin his thoughts about the formulation, asking key evocative questions to elicit commitment to change.

> Therapist – 'Given what you've told me, what do you think you will do next?'
> Kevin – 'I'm going to stop smoking weed during the day and reduce the amount that I buy, but I'm not too sure what else I can do.'
> Therapist – 'You have decided that you are going to reduce the amount that you smoke, and you have also recognised that you may need some help to think about ways of doing this.'

In order to facilitate this the following change plan was developed.

THE CHANGES I WANT TO MAKE ARE:
➤ To stop smoking cannabis
➤ To be able to go out without feeling as scared
➤ To start looking for work.

THE MOST IMPORTANT REASONS I WANT TO MAKE THESE CHANGES ARE:
➤ To stay out of hospital
➤ To feel less paranoid
➤ To think more clearly and improve my memory
➤ To get more enjoyment out of life
➤ To have more money to treat myself.

THE STEPS I PLAN TO TAKE IN CHANGING ARE:
➤ Reduce the amount of cannabis that I buy
➤ Begin by not having a smoke till night time
➤ Avoid spending time with friends who smoke
➤ Identify all the things that I associate with using cannabis and make an effort to avoid them
➤ Work on a plan of gradually increasing my confidence getting out of the house
➤ Speak with my case manager about help to get back into work
➤ Meet regularly with my therapist to look at ways of managing paranoia
➤ Reduce my hypervigilance
➤ Take medication more regularly
➤ Get back in touch with friends who don't smoke
➤ Go fishing with my brother-in-law.

THE WAYS OTHER PEOPLE CAN HELP ME ARE:
➤ My case manager will have ideas about support to get back into work.
➤ I'll go to the gym and other places with a support worker.
➤ My sister has said that I can visit her more often.

I WILL KNOW MY PLAN IS WORKING IF:
➤ I am not smoking cannabis
➤ I am getting out of the house more often
➤ I am feeling more confident in dealing with feelings of vulnerability and paranoia
➤ Other people notice that I'm doing well.

SOME THINGS THAT COULD GET IN THE WAY OF MY PLAN ARE:
➤ Replacing cannabis with alcohol or amphetamine
➤ Boredom
➤ Still feeling paranoid
➤ Slipping back into smoking more often to treat myself
➤ Not wanting to see my family, my case manager, my support worker, my therapist
➤ Spending more time with friends who use cannabis and other substances.

WHAT I WILL DO IF MY PLAN ISN'T WORKING:
➤ Don't give myself a hard time – remind myself that change is difficult and that having slip-ups is common
➤ Request more help to get through difficult times
➤ Go through this plan with my case manager to identify what extra help I may need
➤ Remind myself why I made the change in the first place.

Phase two: moving into action

Kevin began to experiment with reducing his cannabis use. From a baseline of using a £20 bag per day, he reduced his use to a £20 bag per week. Kevin reported that his concentration was improving, that his elder sister was commenting positively on this change and that overall he was feeling less paranoid. Yet, despite this, he reported that he was not going out as often as he would have liked. His case manager struggled, due to staff shortages, to obtain a support worker who could assist Kevin to take part in more social activities. Kevin was also becoming frustrated by the delay in being seen by the team responsible for helping people back into employment. He began to miss appointments with his therapist, and was spending more time with his cannabis-using friends who continued to visit him. Kevin increased his cannabis use leading to him feeling more paranoid and his sister having to contact the crisis team.

The therapist attempted to re-engage with Kevin, making a number of short but frequent visits as in the early stages of therapy. Kevin's ambivalence had returned and it was the task of the therapist to explore this once more by eliciting 'change talk' statements while being careful not to arouse resistance from Kevin. Looking at Kevin's difficulties again further highlighted that his fears were more likely to be evident when tired, bored or experiencing a hangover from recent cannabis use. Intrusive paranoid thoughts of imminent danger, exacerbated by an underlying self-perception that he was weak and vulnerable, led to feelings of anxiety, frustration and low mood, and unhelpful responses including not wanting to go out, being hypervigilant to danger, and smoking more cannabis. This led to a number of disabling consequences such as being socially isolated, increased paranoid thinking, increased risk of hospitalisation and not being able to achieve his cherished values and goals.

Kevin and the therapist spent time reviewing the previous formulation (Figure 11.2) and the change plan. This helped the therapist to discuss Kevin's options in light of his own previously identified change statements. Kevin decided that he was going to work on:
➤ reducing cannabis use once more
➤ reducing hypervigilant behaviours
➤ becoming more active
➤ developing alternative interpretations of intrusive paranoid thoughts.

These then became the focus for a more CBT oriented intervention in the remaining sessions.

After several more months and 26 sessions of therapy in total, Kevin had again reduced his cannabis use. He used cannabis very occasionally and had committed to not buying any for his own personal use. He was working towards getting into some kind of paid employment, had become more socially active with the help of a new support worker and, importantly, was spending more time with his sister and brother-in-law with whom he went fishing. Kevin had reduced his hypervigilant behaviours and he had begun to develop more benign explanations for the intrusive thoughts he experienced.

CONCLUSION

> **KEY POINT 11.6**
>
> Motivational interviewing when integrated with cognitive behavioural therapy is a promising approach to working alongside people experiencing psychosis and substance use problems.

Working alongside individuals experiencing psychosis-substance use problems can present a number of challenges for mental health professionals and it is not surprising that there has been difficulty in developing effective approaches for this population. From our clinical experience, the integrated therapeutic approach described in this chapter shows some cautious promise as a way to build motivation to change substance use while identifying and addressing the difficulties that maintain substance use disorders in psychosis. Integrating MI into recognised CBT approaches for psychosis and substance use can help to strengthen engagement and retention in treatment through the recognition and acceptance of the various aspects of ambivalence expressed by the individual with these difficulties.

REFERENCES

1 Regier DA, Farmer ME, Rae DS, *et al.* Comorbidity of mental disorders with alcohol and other drug abuse: results from the epidemiological catchment area (ECA) Study. *Journal of the American Medical Association.* 1990; **264**: 2511–8.

2 Kessler RC, Crum RM, Warner LA, *et al.* Lifetime co-occurrence of DSM-III-R alcohol abuse and dependence with other psychiatric disorders in the national comorbidity survey. *Archives of General Psychiatry.* 1997; **54**: 313–21.

3 Blanchard JJ, Brown SA, Horan WP, *et al.* Substance use disorders in schizophrenia: review, integration and a proposed model. *Clinical Psychology Review.* 2000; **20**: 207–34.

4 Kavanagh D, McGrath J, Saunders J, *et al.* Substance misuse in patients with schizophrenia: epidemiology and management. *Drugs.* 2002; **62**: 743–55.

5 Todd J, Green G, Harrison M, *et al.* Social exclusion in clients with comorbid mental health and substance use problems. *Social Psychiatry and Psychiatric Epidemiology.* 2004; **39**: 581–7.

6 Coldham EL, Addington J, Addington D. Medication adherence of individuals with a first episode of psychosis. *Acta Psychiatrica Scandinavica.* 2002; **106**: 286–90.

7 Janssen B, Gaebel W, Haerter M, *et al.* Evaluation of factors influencing medication compliance in inpatient treatment of psychotic disorders. *Psychopharmacology.* 2006; **187**: 229–36.

8 Swofford DC, Scheller-Gilkey G, Miller AH, *et al.* Double jeopardy: schizophrenia and substance use. *American Journal of Drug and Alcohol Abuse.* 2000; **26**: 343–53.

9 Menezes PR, Johnson S, Thornicroft G, *et al.* Drug and alcohol problems among individuals with severe mental illnesses in south London. *British Journal of Psychiatry.* 1996; **168**: 612–19.

10 Linszen DH, Dingemans PM, Lenior ME. Cannabis abuse and the course of recent-onset schizophrenic disorders. *Archives of General Psychiatry.* 1994; **51**: 273–9.

11 Cuffel BJ, Shumway M, Chouljian TL, *et al.* A longitudinal study of substance use and community violence in schizophrenia. *Journal of Nervous and Mental Disease.* 1994; **182**: 704–8.

12 Fulwiler C, Grossman H, Forbes C, *et al.* Early onset substance use and community violence by outpatients with chronic mental illness. *Psychiatric Services.* 1997; **48**: 1181–5.

13 Hawton K, Sutton L, Haw C, *et al.* Schizophrenia and suicide: systematic review of risk factors. *British Journal of Psychiatry.* 2005; **187**: 9–20.

14 Kamali M, Kelly L, Gervin M, *et al.* The prevalence of comorbid substance misuse and its influence on suicidal ideation among in-patients with schizophrenia. *Acta Psychiatrica Scandinavica.* 2000; **101**: 452–6.

15 Mueser KT, Drake RE, Sigmon S, *et al.* Psychosocial interventions for adults with severe mental illnesses and co-occurring substance use disorders: a review of specific interventions. *Journal of Dual Diagnosis.* 2005; **1**: 57–82.

16 Drake RE, Mueser KT, Brunette MF, *et al.* A review of treatments for persons with severe mental illness and co-occurring substance use disorder. *Psychiatric Rehabilitation Journal.* 2004; **27**: 360–74.

17 Barrowclough C, Haddock G, Lowens I, *et al.* Psychosis and drug and alcohol problems. In: Baker A, Velleman S, editors . *Clinical Handbook of Co-Existing Mental Health & Drug & Alcohol Problems.* New York, NY: Routledge/Taylor & Francis; 2007.

18 Ziedonis D, Smelson D, Rosenthal RN, *et al.* Improving the care of individuals with schizophrenia and substance use disorders: consensus recommendations. *Journal of Psychiatric Practice.* 2005; **11**: 315–39.

19 Mueser, KT, Drake R. Integrated dual disorder treatment in New Hampshire (USA). In: Graham HL, Copello A, Birchwood MJ, *et al*, editors. *Substance Misuse in Psychosis: approaches to treatment and service delivery.* Chichester: Wiley; 2003.

20 Baker A, Lewin T, Reichler H, *et al.* Evaluation of a motivational interview for substance use within psychiatric in-patient services. *Addiction.* 2002; **97**: 1329–37.

21 Barrowclough C, Haddock G, Tarrier N, *et al.* Randomized controlled trial of motivational interviewing, cognitive behavior therapy, and family intervention for patients with comorbid schizophrenia and substance use disorders. *American Journal of Psychiatry.* 2001; **158**: 1706–13.

22 Barrowclough C, Haddock G, Fitzsimmons M, *et al.* Treatment development for psychosis and co-occurring substance misuse: a descriptive review. *Journal of Mental Health.* 2006; **15**: 619–32.

23 Graeber DA, Moyers TB, Griffith G, *et al.* A pilot study comparing motivational interviewing and an educational intervention in patients with schizophrenia and alcohol use disorders. *Community Mental Health Journal.* 2003; **39**: 189–202.

24 Pilling S, Bebbington P, Kuipers E, *et al.* Psychological treatments in schizophrenia: I. meta-analysis of family intervention and cognitive behaviour therapy. *Psychological Medicine.* 2002; **32**: 763–82.

25 Haddock G, Barrowclough C, Tarrier N, *et al.* Cognitive-behavioural therapy and

motivational intervention for schizophrenia and substance use: 18-month outcomes of a randomised controlled trial. *British Journal of Psychiatry.* 2003; **183**: 418–26.

26 Barrowclough C, Haddock G, Beardmore R, *et al.* Evaluating integrated MI and CBT for people with psychosis and substance misuse: recruitment, retention and sample characteristics of the MIDAS trial. *Addictive Behaviors.* 2009; **34**: 859–66.

27 Weaver T, Madden P, Charles V, *et al.* Comorbidity of substance misuse and mental illness in community mental health and substance misuse services. *British Journal of Psychiatry.* 2003; **183**: 304–13.

28 Chambers RA, Krystal JH, Self DW. A neurobiological basis for substance abuse comorbidity in schizophrenia. *Biological Psychiatry.* 2001; **50**: 71–83.

29 Verdoux H, Gindre C, Sorbara F, *et al.* Effects of cannabis psychosis vulnerability in daily life: an experience sampling test study. *Psychological Medicine.* 2003; **33**: 23–32.

30 Drake R, Osher FC, Wallach MA. Alcohol use and abuse in schizophrenia: a prospective community study. *Journal of Nervous and Mental Disease.* 1989; **17**: 408–14.

31 Neuchterlein KH, Dawson M. A heuristic vulnerability/stress model of schizophrenic episodes. *Schizophrenia Bulletin.* 1984; **10**: 300–12.

32 Gregg L, Barrowclough C, Haddock G. Reasons for increased substance use in psychosis. *Clinical Psychology Review.* 2007; **27**: 494–510.

33 Kavanagh DJ, Waghorn G, Jenner L, *et al.* Demographic and clinical correlates of comorbid substance use disorders in psychosis: multivariate analyses from an epidemiological sample. *Schizophrenia Research.* 2004; **66**: 115–24.

34 Patkar AA, Alexander RC, Lundy A, *et al.* Changing patterns of illicit substance use among schizophrenic patients. *American Journal of Addiction.* 1999; **8**: 65–71.

35 Khantzian EJ. The self-medication hypothesis of substance use disorders: a reconsideration and recent applications. *Harvard Review of Psychiatry.* 1997; **4**: 231–44.

36 Gregg L, Haddock G, Barrowclough C. Self-reported reasons for substance use in schizophrenia: a Q methodological investigation. *Mental Health and Substance Use: Dual Diagnosis.* 2009; **2**: 24–39.

37 Teesson M, Hall W, Lynskey M, *et al.* Alcohol- and drug-use disorders in Australia: implications of the national survey of mental health and well-being, *Australia and New Zealand Journal of Psychiatry.* 2000; **34**: 206–13.

38 Marlatt GA, Gordon JR. *Relapse Prevention: maintenance strategies in the treatment of addictive behaviours.* New York: Guilford Press; 1985.

39 Conrod PJ, Stewart SH. A critical look at dual-focused cognitive-behavioural treatments for comorbid substance use and psychiatric disorders: strengths, limitations, and future directions. *Journal of Cognitive Psychotherapy.* 2005; **19**: 261–84.

40 Carey KB, Carey MP. Reasons for drinking among psychiatric outpatients: relationship to drinking patterns. *Psychology of Addictive Behaviours.* 1995; **9**: 251–7.

41 Lobbana F, Barrowclough C, Jeffery S, *et al.* Understanding factors influencing substance use in people with recent onset psychosis: a qualitative study. *Social Science and Medicine.* 2010; **70**: 1141–7.

42 Bellack AS, DiClemente CC. Treating substance abuse among patients with schizophrenia. *Psychiatric Services.* 1999; **50**: 75–80.

43 Miller WR, Rollnick S. *Motivational Interviewing: preparing people for change.* 2nd ed. New York: Guilford Press; 2002.

44 Arkowitz H, Burke BL. Motivational interviewing as an integrative framework for the treatment of depression. In: Arkowitz H, Westra HA, Miller WR, *et al. Motivational Interviewing in the Treatment of Psychological Problems.* New York: Guilford Press; 2008.

45 Available at: www.motivationalinterviewing.org (accessed 7 October 2010).

46 Miller WR. Motivational interviewing with problem drinkers. *Behavioural Psychotherapy.* 1983; **11**: 147–72.

47 Amrhein PC. How does motivational interviewing work? What client talk reveals. *Journal of Cognitive Psychotherapy.* 2004; **18**: 323–36.

48 Rollnick S, Miller WR, Butler CC. *Motivational Interviewing in Health Care: helping patients change behavior.* New York: Guilford Press; 2008.

49 McCracken SG, Corrigan PW. Motivational interviewing for medication adherence in individuals with schizophrenia. In: Arkowitz H, Westra AH, Miller WR, *et al. Motivational Interviewing in the Treatment of Psychological Problems.* New York: Guilford Press; 2008.

50 Martino S, Carroll KM, Kostas D, *et al.* Dual diagnosis motivational interviewing: a modification of motivational interviewing for substance-abusing patients with psychotic disorders. *Journal of Substance Abuse Treatment.* 2002; **23**: 297–308.

51 Handmaker N, Packard M, Conforti K. Motivational interviewing in the treatment of dual disorders. In: Miller WR, Rollnick S, editors. *Motivational Interviewing: preparing people for change.* 2nd ed. New York: Guilford press; 2002.

52 Carey KB. Substance use reduction in the context of outpatient psychiatric treatment: a collaborative, motivational harm reduction approach. *Community Mental Health Journal.* 1996; **32**: 291–306.

53 Ziedonis DM, Fisher W. Motivation-based assessment and treatment of substance abuse in patients with schizophrenia. *Directions in Psychiatry.* 1996; **16**: 1–8.

54 Martino S, Moyers TB. Motivational Interviewing with dually diagnosed patients. In: Arkowitz H, Westra AH, Miller WR, *et al. Motivational Interviewing in the Treatment of Psychological Problems.* New York: Guilford Press; 2008.

55 Haddock G, Tarrier N. Assessment and formulation in the cognitive behavioural treatment of psychosis. In: Tarrier N, Wells A, Haddock G, editors, *Treating Complex Cases: the cognitive behavioural approach.* Chichester: Guilford Press; 1998.

56 Morrison AP, editor. *A Casebook of Cognitive Therapy for Psychosis.* New York: Taylor & Francis; 2002.

57 National Institute for Health and Clinical Excellence. *Core Interventions in the Treatment and Management of Schizophrenia in Primary and Secondary Care (update): NICE Guideline CG82.* London: NIHCE; 2009. Available at: http://guidance.nice.org.uk/CG82 (accessed 7 October 2010).

58 Westra HA, Dozois DJA. Integrating motivational interviewing into the treatment of anxiety. In: Arkowitz H, Westra AH, Miller WR, *et al. Motivational Interviewing in the Treatment of Psychological Problems.* New York: Guilford Press; 2008.

59 Arkowitz H, Miller WR, Westra HA, *et al.* Motivational interviewing in the treatment of psychological problems: conclusions and future directions. In: Arkowitz H, Westra AH, Miller WR, *et al. Motivational Interviewing in the Treatment of Psychological Problems.* New York: Guilford Press; 2008.

60 Martino S, Moyers TB. 'What's Important in My Life': the personal goals and values card sorting task for individuals with schizophrenia. 2006. Available at: http://casaa.unm.edu/inst/Values%20Card%20Sorting%20Task%20for%20Individuals%20with%20Schizophrenia.pdf (accessed 7 October 2010).

61 Barrowclough C, Nothard S, Haddock G, *et al.* MiCBT: *An Integrated Psychological Therapy for People with Psychosis and Substance Use: therapy manual.* Manchester: University of Manchester; 2008. Available on request from author.

TO LEARN MORE

- www.motivationalinterview.org (accessed 24 January 2011).
- www.midastrial.ac.uk (accessed 24 January 2011).
- Baker A, Velleman S, editors. *Clinical Handbook of Co-existing Mental Health & Drug & Alcohol Problems.* New York: Routledge/Taylor & Francis; 2007.
- Miller WR, Rollnick S. *Motivational Interviewing: preparing people for change.* 2nd ed. New York: Guilford Press; 2002.
- Rollnick S, Miller WR, Butler CC. *Motivational Interviewing in Health Care: helping patients change behavior.* New York: Guilford Press; 2008.
- Arkowitz H, Westra AH, Miller WR, *et al.* Motivational Interviewing in the Treatment of Psychological Problems. New York: Guilford Press; 2008.

CHAPTER 12

Cognitive behavioural integrated treatment (C-BIT)

Derek Tobin

PRE-READING EXERCISE 12.1 (ANSWERS ON P. 186)

> **Time: 15 minutes**
> - What is your understanding of integrated treatment?
> - What barriers do you think there may be to the implementation of integrated treatment?
> - What skills do you think staff in mental health services require when working with drug/alcohol use?

INTRODUCTION

Working with people who experience mental health–substance use problems can pose challenges for professionals due to the often complex needs of these individuals. The UK *Dual Diagnosis Good Practice Guide* advocates mainstreaming/integrated treatment where individuals have their mental health and substance use needs addressed concurrently.[1] It can be difficult for professionals to provide integrated services if they have not received appropriate training to enhance their confidence and skills. Integrated treatment advocates a stage-wise treatment approach, which matches interventions to the individual's stage of engagement.[2,3] The effective implementation of integrated treatment is, therefore, dependent on professionals having the skills to deliver a range of interventions that are tailored to the needs of the individual. This chapter describes the development and implementation of cognitive behavioural integrated treatment (C-BIT) within Birmingham and Solihull Mental Health Foundation Trust (BSMHFT), UK.

BACKGROUND

The first stage in the development of C-BIT involved identifying local need through prevalence surveys and staff training and support needs surveys. The prevalence survey identified that 24% (324) of people with a diagnosis of severe and enduring mental health problems within mental health and substance use services had used drugs/alcohol problematically in the previous 12 months.[4] The training and support needs survey identified that professionals felt that it was within their remit to work with individuals experiencing mental health–substance use problems. However, they felt that they did not receive appropriate training, support, information and supervision to do this effectively.[5] The results of these surveys posed two questions:

1　How should services be configured to address mental health and substance use?
2　What should the model of intervention be?

As the trust already had a range of mental health and substance use services – that is, inpatient units, assertive outreach teams (AOT), early intervention service (EIS), crisis teams, community mental health teams (CMHTs) and community drug teams (CDTs) – it was decided not to have a separate mental health–substance use service that worked with a separate caseload as this would provide limited service accessibility based on local prevalence. A service that could work across teams to enhance confidence and skills through training and support was agreed as being more inclusive. This led to the development of an integrated treatment philosophy and to the development of C-BIT as a model of intervention. C-BIT was developed within the COMPASS programme and evaluated in five AOT services.[6]

COGNITIVE BEHAVIOURAL INTEGRATED TREATMENT MODEL

C-BIT is a manualised treatment model designed to enhance the confidence and skills of professionals to work collaboratively alongside individuals. The focus of C-BIT is to promote and maintain behaviour change in problematic drug/alcohol use and to facilitate the development of alternative strategies to enable service users to self-manage their mental health and substance use. C-BIT is, therefore, a structured but flexible cognitive behavioural treatment designed to either stand alone or be used as part of a larger programme of organisational change in the development of a service philosophy of integrated treatment.

　　C-BIT is based on core treatment components to enable professionals to provide a range of evidence-based interventions when working alongside individuals experiencing mental health–substance use problems. The treatment components consist of assessment and four treatment phases:

1　engagement and building motivation to change
2　negotiating behaviour change
3　early relapse prevention
4　relapse prevention (*see* Book 4, Chapter 13; Book 6, Chapters 15 and 16).

There are two further treatment phases, which concentrate on skills building and working with families and social networks. Treatment phases are aligned with the service-user stage of engagement.[7] This helps professionals to match interventions to the person's treatment phase, thus enhancing engagement and promoting a more collaborative relationship (*see* Table 12.1).

TABLE 12.1 Treatment phases

Phase	Goal	C-BIT interventions
Engagement	To establish a working alliance with the individual and be able to discuss alcohol/drug use and any problems it may be causing	**Treatment phase 1** • Strategies to increase engagement • How to put substance use on the agenda • Building motivation to change • Re-evaluating substance-related beliefs • Dealing with resistance • Identifying social networks supportive of change • Finance management
Negotiating behaviour change	To develop the individual's awareness of problems associated with alcohol/drug use and build motivation to change	**Treatment phase 2** • Identifying harm-reduction goals • Working on resistance to goal setting • Behavioural experiments • Identifying activities of interest • Building social networks supportive of change • Increasing awareness of problematic links between mental health and substance use
Early relapse prevention	To help individual further reduce alcohol/drug use and, if possible, attain abstinence	**Treatment phase 3** • Formulating cognitive model of substance use problems • Relapse prevention: helping the individual manage substance use • Relapse prevention: including social network members • Coping with cravings • Relapse prevention for substance use and links to mental health
Relapse prevention/ management	To maintain awareness that relapse could happen and to extend recovery to other areas (e.g. mental health, social, relationships, work)	**Treatment phase 4** • Identifying a signature to psychotic relapse and role of substance use • Developing a comprehensive relapse prevention/management plan • Using a comprehensive relapse/ management plan.

Each treatment phase includes a range of interventions, including cognitive and motivational enhancement techniques (*see* Book 4, Chapters 6, 7, 9 and 10).

COGNITIVE TECHNIQUES

Cognitive strategies within C-BIT focus on substance-related beliefs, cognitive distortions and behavioural experiments to promote change. The cognitive model of substance use problems suggests that positive substance-related beliefs are central to the maintenance of a problematic cycle of substance use.[8] For example, an individual may believe that:

➤ 'Cannabis is the only thing that stops my voices.'
➤ 'Alcohol makes me chilled out and more sociable.'

As these beliefs become reinforced through ongoing substance use, individuals may feel that they can self-manage their mental health problems through substance use.

In order to engage the individual in a process of change, it is important to target substance-related beliefs to facilitate the development of alternative beliefs and promote a change in self-confidence.

MOTIVATIONAL ENHANCEMENT

Motivational techniques are used to enhance engagement primarily when individuals are in the engagement phase – techniques are adapted from motivational interviewing.[9] When people are in the engagement phase they may, for example, be ambivalent about change and make statements like: 'It's up to me if I use crack cocaine or not. I don't want to talk to you about it.'

At this stage, looking at advantages/disadvantages of use may be an appropriate intervention to enhance motivation.

Through these processes C-BIT aims to encourage professionals to take a long-term optimistic approach to working with people, and to recognise that change can be difficult and should be encouraged and supported.

APPLICATION OF COGNITIVE BEHAVIOURAL INTEGRATED TREATMENT IN PRACTICE

The application of C-BIT (within BSMHFT) is facilitated by the COMPASS programme. COMPASS programme professionals provide training and clinical input to mental health teams to enable professionals to integrate C-BIT into clinical practice. Training is provided to whole teams and focuses on the:

➤ assertive outreach team
➤ early intervention service
➤ homeless team
➤ forensic inpatient unit.

Following training, teams receive one clinical day per week from a COMPASS programme professional. The function of the COMPASS programme professionals in these teams is to facilitate the implementation of skills learned in training and to enhance the confidence and skills of the professional through the following:

➤ **Joint working**: Professionals identify people they are working with for whom joint clinical work would be helpful in terms of assessment, formulation and treatment planning. This usually focuses on people who may be more difficult to engage and present as ambivalent in addressing their substance use.

➤ **Supervision/consultation**: Supervision is provided on both a team and an individual basis. Team supervision is facilitated through monthly case discussions facilitated by a COMPASS professional. Professionals in the teams can receive further support through individual supervision and informal consultation.

➤ **Ongoing training**: C-BIT training is provided annually to new staff in EIS, AOT and the homeless team to ensure that the majority of the teams remain trained. Top-up training sessions are also provided within the teams.

EVALUATION

The C-BIT treatment trial was carried out in five local AOTs and addressed two key questions:

1 Can integrated treatment be achieved within existing AOTs?
2 Can integrated treatment demonstrate positive outcomes for individuals?

Integration of C-BIT was assessed through clinical sessions, case notes and team meetings. Impact on individuals was assessed by:

➤ psychiatric symptoms
➤ engagement
➤ amount of substances used
➤ conviction in substance-related beliefs.

Results demonstrated that integrated treatment could be achieved within mainstream mental health teams. This was identified through the positive impact C-BIT training had on the confidence and skills of the professional (which was maintained over time), increased ability to implement C-BIT interventions and a shift in the philosophy of teams. Individuals showed positive engagement in treatment and a reduction in alcohol consumption.[6] Impact was not as significant on cannabis use and this has resulted in a study on staff perception of cannabis through the COMPASS programme research group.

The remainder of this chapter will focus on a case study to illustrate some of the issues discussed so far. The name and details of the individual discussed have been changed to maintain confidentiality. It is important to note that the work identified in this case study was carried out over a period of months, and highlights the need to take a long-term approach.

Case study 12.1: John

John (28) is under the care of an AOT. He has a history of schizophrenia and problematic cannabis use. John has a supportive family and has regular contact with them. His substance use was an important part of his life and he believed that it provided him with a social network where he felt accepted. John was engaged with the AOT, having his depot medication fortnightly. As John experienced a relapse in his mental health he started to disengage from the team. His substance use became chaotic and he became paranoid and avoided contact with his family. There was an increase in John's voices, which were derogatory towards him and made his behaviour erratic. Although the team attempted to remain engaged with John, he was admitted to hospital. During his relapse John had been ambivalent about discussing his substance use with the team, but prior to discharge from hospital he agreed to work with the team who have all had C-BIT training and are supported in its implementation through a professional from the COMPASS programme.

Assessment

Cognitive behavioural integrated treatment assessment consists of a semi-structured clinical interview that includes:

➤ identifying current use including reasons for use; identifying substance-related beliefs, reasons for use and effects/difficulties associated with use
➤ taking a personal drug/alcohol history and developing a time line of life events leading up to current presentation
➤ assessing the links between substance use and mental health.

Information gathered through the assessment is used to develop a formulation that guides interventions collaboratively with the individual.

In developing the formulation there are three important questions to consider:
1 What are the individual's presenting difficulties?
2 How did their difficulties develop?
3 What are the maintaining factors?

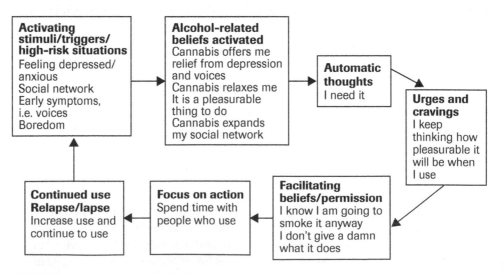

FIGURE 12.1 John's problematic cycle of use

Following assessment, a formulation was developed with John to identify his persisting cycle of problematic substance use (Figure 12.1).

The main issues for John were boredom, his social network and distressing symptoms. These high-risk situations triggered John's beliefs that 'cannabis relaxes me and is a pleasurable thing to do'. He described persistent thoughts about the outcome expectancy of cannabis ('I keep thinking how pleasurable it will be'). These thoughts led John to minimise the consequences ('I don't give a damn what it does'). He used and continued to use increasing amounts. To look at tipping the balance in favour of change, motivational strategies were utilised.

Building motivation to change: cognitive behavioural integrated treatment – phase one

Although John had engaged in the assessment process and in identifying his cycle of use, he remained ambivalent about addressing his cannabis use and the impact it was having on his mental health. To engage John in discussing this further, an advantages/disadvantages analysis was carried out. The purpose of this was to give John the opportunity to identify the good things associated with his cannabis use as well as any concerns (Table 12.2). When doing this exercise it is important that professionals facilitate the process and are not prescriptive in their approach.

TABLE 12.2 Advantages/disadvantages analysis

	ADVANTAGES (FOR)	DISADVANTAGES (AGAINST)
SHORT TERM	• Cannabis makes me feel good • I love the buzz • Cannabis eases my voices • Cannabis gives me a good social network	• Cannabis can make me paranoid • Cannabis makes me anxious • Smoking cannabis causes problems with my family • I feel less motivated when I smoke cannabis
LONG TERM	• I enjoy the buzz and good feeling	• Nothing will change for me • Will lose my family.

Self-motivational statements could include:

➤ **Concern**: 'Cannabis makes me less motivated to do things like going to college and getting on with my life.'
➤ **Intent to change**: 'I need to cut down my cannabis use or things will not change for me.'

Although John was able to identify disadvantages to his use, his focus prior to this exercise was primarily the fact that he believed that the advantages outweighed the disadvantages. Through this exercise, John identified that his main concern was the impact that his cannabis use was having on his family relationships. This enhanced his motivation to change. To further enhance John's motivation we completed a decisional balance exercise.

Decisional balance

The decisional balance exercise enables individuals to focus on the pros and cons of making changes in substance use. This helps to identify the potential benefits that change will bring as well as highlight the obstacles to change and the cognitive distortions that may contribute to this. *See* Table 12.3 for the decisional balance John identified.

TABLE 12.3 Behaviour: cut down cannabis use

	'PROS' (FOR)	'CONS' (AGAINST)
SHORT TERM	• I will be more motivated to do other things like college • Family relationships will be better • My mental health will be more stable • I will have more money to spend on going out, buying clothes	• I will lose my social network • I will not be able to relax • I will feel more stressed • I will miss the buzz from cannabis
LONG TERM	• I will feel healthier • I will be able to get a job	• I will miss the buzz.

Self-motivational statements might include:
➤ **Concern**: 'My cannabis use is making me less motivated to do things and get on with my life.'
➤ **Intent to change**: 'I need to cut down my cannabis as it is causing problems with my family.'

John was able to identify that the main reasons for change were that his mental health would be more stable and that he would have better family relationships, which were very important to him. By focusing on areas against change we were able to identify some cognitive distortions that may have prevented John from making further changes. For example, John believed that he would lose his social network. But when this belief was discussed, it became clear to John that although he might lose *some* people in his social network he could focus on spending more time with people in his social network who did not use cannabis. This would enhance his ability to develop a social network supportive of change. John was able to focus on this; however, he remained concerned that he would not be able to cut down his cannabis use.

Negotiating behaviour change: cognitive behavioural integrated treatment – phase two

Although John managed to reduce his cannabis use, he remained concerned that he would not be able to make further reductions. To enhance John's engagement and confidence in his ability to make changes, we worked collaboratively to develop a behavioural experiment to test out John's thought that he would not be able to go for one day without using cannabis (Table 12.4).

TABLE 12.4 Lessons learned

Experiment	Prediction	Potential obstacles	Strategies to overcome obstacles	Outcome of experiment
Not to smoke cannabis for one day	I will feel anxious and uptight	My friends will encourage me to use	Arrange to spend time with friend who does not use	Felt anxious but spent time with family and went out with friend
		Agitation will get the better of me	Visit family	It was hard but I did it

The lesson learned might include: 'It was difficult to do but I showed myself that I can do it'.

John's main concern was that he would feel anxious and would not be able to resist using when his friends came round. Looking at strategies to overcome these obstacles helped to enhance John's confidence in making changes. He agreed that he would arrange to spend time with friends who did not use and to spend some time with his family. This felt achievable to John and something that he felt able to try. Although he found it difficult he could see that identifying alternatives to cannabis use enabled him to achieve further harm-reduction goals.

Early relapse prevention: cognitive behavioural integrated treatment – phase three

As work progressed with John, he made significant changes in his cannabis use and engaged in structured work to address both his mental health and his substance use. At this stage early relapse prevention was introduced. The purpose of this was to enable John to identify areas that would help self-management of his mental health and substance use and to maintain changes already made. John's problematic cycle of use was reviewed as this formed the basis of a relapse plan for substance use (Figure 12.2).

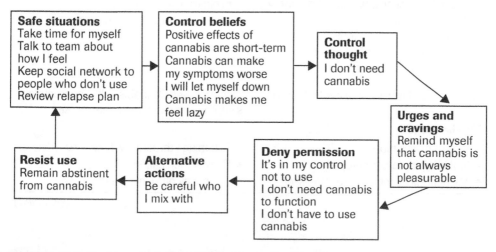

FIGURE 12.2 Review of John's problematic cycle of use

Through this process, John was able to identify alternatives to his problematic cycle that would help to minimise his risk of relapse. To ensure that this was a meaningful exercise, work was carried out to ensure that John could identify meaningful alternatives to his trigger situations. We also worked together to re-evaluate John's positive substance-related beliefs. This involved John identifying evidence that supported his beliefs and evidence that did not. It enabled him to identify substance-related beliefs that were more realistic to him in terms of the impact cannabis had on his mental health and daily functioning.

Relapse prevention/management: cognitive behavioural integrated treatment – phase four

Over the course of working with John, his goals changed from wanting to cut down his cannabis use (to what he felt would be non-problematic use) to abstinence. Working with John on his self-identified harm-reduction goals helped to increase his confidence to make changes. Initially abstinence had seemed like a goal that was not achievable. John made a very good recovery in his mental health following his hospital admission and was willing to engage in mental health relapse prevention based on the 'back in the saddle model'.[10] This involved reviewing John's recent relapse and getting him to identify the early, middle and late stages. Substance-related beliefs and the function of substance use at each stage of relapse were included to ensure an integrated relapse-management plan that included both mental health and substance use (Table 12.5).

TABLE 12.5 Relapse signatures and drill

Relapse signature	Relapse drill
Early stage	
• Start to believe that I have a special role in the world • Avoid contact with family • Keep things secret because I do not want to go to hospital • Symptoms are not distressing at this stage and make me feel good • Increase cannabis use	• Talk to family/team • Review relapse plan • Review relapse plan for substance to minimise risk of relapse • Discuss medication with team
Belief. Cannabis will make me feel good	*Control belief.* Cannabis will exacerbate my symptoms and make me feel worse
Middle stage	
• Isolate myself more • Not sleeping/eating properly • My actions become more impulsive	• Talk things through with care coordinator • Review medication • Try to stay off/minimise drug use

(continued)

Relapse signature	Relapse drill
• Mood fluctuates at times, feel high then feel low • Don't want to discuss things with people including family and team • Increase my cannabis use further	• Increase visits from team • Consider spending time in respite
Belief: Cannabis will make me feel better and stabilise my mood	*Control belief:* Cannabis makes me more likely to make decisions I regret
Late stage	
• Not bothered what happens to me • I will end up in hospital anyway • Feel powerless • Feel more agitated • Wear inappropriate clothes • Thoughts racing; floods of emotions going through my head	• Increased visits from team • Contact with home treatment • Minimise cannabis use to prevent exacerbation of symptoms • Consider home treatment/hospital admission • Focus on safe situations, spend time with supportive social network members
Belief: Cannabis will slow me down and give me relief	*Control belief:* Cannabis does not always help me and can make my symptoms worse.

CONCLUSION

This chapter has given an overview of the C-BIT model and its clinical application. Cognitive behavioural integrated treatment provides professionals with a framework to work alongside people in a flexible but structured way, focusing on evidence-based interventions. The approach can be used as a stand-alone model or as a process to enhance organisational change as outlined. Training is essential to philosophy change within mental health services and to enhance confidence and skills. The provision of inclusive and accessible services is crucial to enhance engagement and positive experience of services. C-BIT aims to address these issues through an integrated approach that makes mental health–substance use the responsibility of all mental health and substance use services.

POST-READING EXERCISE 12.1 (ANSWERS ON P. 187)

Time: 10 minutes
- How would you describe the C-BIT model?
- How is C-BIT applied in practice?
- How can C-BIT contribute to organisational change for people experiencing mental health–substance use problems?

REFERENCES

1 Department of Health. Mental *Health Policy Implementation Guide: dual diagnosis good practice guide.* London: Department of Health; 2002.

2 Graham HL, Copello A, Birchwood M, *et al. Cognitive Behavioural Integrated Treatment (C-BIT): a treatment manual for substance misuse in people with severe mental health problems.* West Sussex: John Wiley & Sons; 2004.

3 Mueser KT, Noordsy DL, Drake RE, *et al. Integrated Treatment for Dual Disorders: effective intervention for severe mental illness and substance abuse.* New York: Guilford Press; 2003.

4 Graham HL, Maslin J, Copello A, *et al.* Drug and alcohol problems among individuals with severe mental health problems in an inner city area of the UK. *Social Psychiatry and Psychiatric Epidemiology.* 2001; **36**: 448–55.

5 Maslin J, Graham HL, Cawley MA, *et al.* Combined severe mental health and substance use problems: what are the training and support needs of staff working with this client group? *Journal of Mental Health.* 2001; **10**: 131–40.

6 Graham HL, Copello A, Birchwood M, *et al.* A preliminary evaluation of integrated treatment for co-existing substance use and severe mental health problems: impact on teams and service users. *Journal of Mental Health.* 2006; **15**: 577–91.

7 Mueser K, Drake RE, Noordsy DL. Integrated mental health and substance abuse treatment for severe psychiatric disorders. *Journal of Practical Psychiatry and Behavioural Health.* 1998; **4**: 129–39.

8 Beck AT, Wright FD, Newman CF, *et al. Cognitive Therapy of Substance Abuse.* New York: Guilford Press; 1993.

9 Miller W, Rollnick. S. *Motivational Interviewing: preparing people for change.* London: Guilford Press; 1991.

10 Plaistow J, Birchwood M. *Back in the Saddle: early intervention service.* North Birmingham Mental Health Trust. Unpublished manual; 1996.

TO LEARN MORE

- Baker A, Velleman R, editors. *Clinical Handbook of Co-existing Mental Health and Drug and Alcohol Problems.* East Sussex: Routledge; 2007.
- Graham H, Copello A, Birchwood M, *et al,* editors. *Substance Misuse in Psychosis: approaches to treatment and service delivery.* West Sussex: John Wiley & Sons; 2003.

ANSWERS TO PRE-READING EXERCISE 12.1

- Integrated treatment is a process that enables mental health and substance use to be addressed within existing mental health and substance use services. This promotes a holistic approach and prevents individuals being passed among services.
- Barriers may include lack of training and support for professionals and the lack of clearly defined organisational responsibilities.
- Professionals need to have good awareness of substance use and the impact on mental health. The ability to assess, formulate and provide interventions based on the individual's stage of engagement are important to promote effective working.

ANSWERS TO POST-READING EXERCISE 12.1

- C-BIT is a structured but flexible cognitive behavioural treatment approach that provides a range of evidence-based interventions tailored to individual need and stage of engagement.
- C-BIT can be used as a stand-alone model or to enhance organisational change. Treatment interventions are based on assessment and formulation. This guides interventions to the individual's stage of change. Interventions are delivered using a flexible approach based on individualised needs.
- C-BIT can be integrated within existing services to enhance a service philosophy of integrated treatment.

CHAPTER 13

Pharmacological management

Cynthia MA Geppert and Kenneth Minkoff

PRE-READING EXERCISE 13.1

Time: 10 minutes
Read the case study then consider how you would respond to Jack's request.

Case study
Jack (40) has a history of long-standing bipolar disorder and alcohol dependence; he discontinued lithium six months ago, and relapsed to alcohol one week ago due to an emerging depression. Over the weekend he became intoxicated, and developed suicidal ideation. He calls the co-occurring disorders clinic on Monday saying he has been sober one day and needs medication for depression.

Comment
Take a good history then restart the lithium and reinforce the need for continued sobriety.

After you finish the chapter return to reflect on your initial response

BACKGROUND

People experiencing mental health–substance use disorders represent a clinically complex and professionally challenging but rewarding group. Research shows that these individuals have poorer outcomes (including higher risk of morbidity and mortality) despite higher treatment costs.[1]

KEY POINT 13.1

Mental health–substance use disorders are an expectation not an exception.

According to the principles of the Comprehensive Continuous Integrated System of

Care (CCISC), all sectors of the healthcare system (all programmes and all professionals, including prescribers) must develop organised competency in providing integrated services to individuals experiencing mental health–substance use disorders, within their existing resources.[2]

SELF-ASSESSMENT EXERCISE 13.1

Time: 10 minutes
- In your current practice setting, can you identify individuals experiencing mental health–substance use disorders?
- What barriers to providing high-quality care can you list?

Providing information and guidance for best practice in using medications to treat mental health–substance use disorders is the intent of this chapter; it will present general principles and specific recommendations.

All professionals, especially prescribers, should anticipate that any person seen for a psychopharmacological evaluation for a mental illness may also have one or more substance use disorders, and any person seen for a psychopharmacologic or medical evaluation for substance use disorder may have a mental health condition. This expectation is essential not only for organising the process of initial assessment but also as a framework for designing strategies of continuing care.

There is a growing assortment of effective and safe medications available to treat opioid and alcohol dependence as well as a number of agents that may be useful for cocaine dependence.[3] There are also several beneficial pharmaceutical options for the treatment of nicotine dependence, which space will not permit us to discuss. The reader is referred to several excellent references on this topic.[4,5]

SEVEN GENERAL PRINCIPLES

BOX 13.1 General principles

---

1 Mental health–substance use disorders are an expectation not an exception.
2 Successful treatment is based on empathic, hopeful, integrated and continuing relationships.
3 Case management and clinical care must be properly balanced with empathic detachment, opportunities for empowerment and choice, contracting and contingent learning.
4 When mental illness and substance use coexist, each disorder is 'primary', requiring integrated, properly matched, diagnosis-specific treatment of equal intensity.
5 Both serious mental illness and substance dependence disorders are primary bio-psychosocial conditions that can be treated in the context of a 'disease and recovery' model, with interventions matched to phase of recovery and stage of change for each disorder.
6 Treatment must be individualised, using a structured approach to determine the best treatment, based on:

a diagnosis
b acuity
c severity
d disability
e phase of recovery
f stage of change for each disorder.
7 Similarly, there is no one correct psychopharmacological or other approach to individuals experiencing mental health–substance use disorders.

SUCCESSFUL TREATMENT RELATIONSHIPS

A *sine qua non* of the effective practice of both the art and the science of medication treatment is the ability of the professional to welcome individuals who may have active mental health–substance use disorders to identify their disorders accurately, and to establish an empathic, hopeful, integrated, and continuous relationship focused on simultaneous care of both disorders.

Emerging research supports individualised treatment that matches the intervention to the person's type and level of severity of both illnesses, as the most successful. One such model is the 'four-quadrant model' (Table 13.1).

TABLE 13.1 Four-quadrant model

Both: high severity	Mental illness: low severity Substance use disorder: high severity **(substance dependence)**
Mental illness: high severity Substance use disorder: low severity **(substance abuse)**	Both: low severity

The quadrants are based on an assignment of either low or high severity for each disorder. Psychopharmacological treatments can also be adapted to, and adopted for, the particular combination of disorder type and severity. For example, individuals with serious and persistent mental illnesses such as schizophrenia or bipolar disorder are most likely to be considered high priority for engaging in continuing medication treatment located in the mental health system. The acuity and severity of the substance use disorder (active versus remission, abuse or dependence) will also influence the pharmacological decision-making process. It is particularly important when considering pharmacological options to distinguish substance *abuse* as a biobehavioural disorder involving poor choices from substance *dependence* that is a brain disease.

KEY POINT 13.2

The threshold for use of substances may be lower in individuals with serious mental illness so it is important for prescribers to clearly identify use for dependence when making medication decisions, especially in relation to addictive drugs like opioids and benzodiazepines.

CASE MANAGEMENT AND CLINICAL CARE

Learning is a key feature of care for mental health–substance use disorders; the pharmacological relationship must strive to balance the ongoing need for medication management with opportunities for *contingent learning* in the management of both mental health and substance use conditions; for example:

➤ negotiating choice of medications, routes, timing and quantity as well as duration of treatment and manner of cessation

➤ mutual acceptance by professional and individual of the trial-and-error nature of prescribing.

For treatment negotiations like these to result in productive growth, the one thing that must not be *contingent* is maintenance of the therapeutic relationship (*see* Book 4, Chapter 2).

MENTAL ILLNESS AND SUBSTANCE USE ARE EACH PRIMARY DISORDERS

Earlier philosophies of care prioritised one disorder over the other; the presumption of modern models is that when two disorders co-occur, *both* are primary. Pharmacological interventions are designed to maximise the outcome of the two primary disorders through adherence to the following maxims.

➤ For most diagnosed psychiatric disorders, the individual receives the most clinically effective evidence-based psychopharmacological treatment available regardless of the type or status of the comorbid substance use disorder.

➤ Medications that may be used for treatment of substance use disorders (such as naltrexone for alcohol dependence) can be used as ancillary and adjunctive to a comprehensive programme of addiction recovery, and should be considered when appropriate for the substance use disorder, even in the presence of a comorbid psychiatric disorder.

➤ There are no 'magic bullets' for the treatment of mental health–substance use disorders. There is evidence suggesting that some commonly used psychiatric medications may result in modest improvement for certain addictive disorders. For example, the use of clozapine in co-occurring substance dependence,[6] selective serotonin reuptake inhibitors (SSRIs) in type II alcoholics,[7] and mood stabilisers such as topiramate and valproate in alcohol dependence.

BOTH DISORDERS CAN BE TREATED IN A 'DISEASE AND RECOVERY MODEL'

A recovery orientation capitalising on strengths and resilience is increasingly recognised as the most promising model for the treatment of both disorders. Pharmacological practice will depend on the individual's phase of recovery and stage of change (Table 13.2 – *see* Book 4, Chapters 6 and 7). For example, a professional may provide continuing antipsychotic treatment for psychosis and motivational engagement interventions for an individual experiencing schizophrenia and alcohol dependence, who is in the late action stage for his schizophrenia, but in precontemplation or contemplation for alcohol dependence.

TABLE 13.2 Recovering phases and stage of change

Four phases of recovery	Stages of change
Acute stabilisation: detoxification	
Motivational enhancement/engagement	**Precontemplation, contemplation, preparation**
Prolonged stabilisation: active treatment or relapse prevention	**Early and late action**
Rehabilitation and recovery	**Maintenance**

THERE IS NO ONE CORRECT PSYCHOPHARMACOLOGICAL APPROACH TO INDIVIDUALS EXPERIENCING MENTAL HEALTH–SUBSTANCE USE DISORDERS

Clinical interventions, including prescribing of medications, must be matched to the individual's specific diagnoses, degree of acuity, impairment or severity of each disorder, phase of recovery and stage of change.

CLINICAL PRACTICE GUIDELINES
Welcoming

➤ A welcoming approach in which the prescriber views all individuals as high risk and high priority, deserving empathy, hope and integrated continuous treatment, is the most successful.

Access

➤ It is now well recognised (compared with what was taught in previous years) that there should be no requirement for an arbitrary length of sobriety before assessing comorbid psychiatric disorders or prescribing indicated medications.

KEY POINT 13.3

There should not be a requirement for an arbitrary duration of sobriety preceding a comorbid psychiatric evaluation.

➤ Any individual able to participate in a clinical interview, whatever his/her state of intoxication or withdrawal, should be assessed as promptly as possible.
➤ Medical and psychiatric acuity and risk factors for suicide, violence and inability to care for self should determine the urgency of immediate psychopharmacological evaluation and intervention.

➤ It is prudent to maintain current non-addictive psychotropic regimens during detoxification and early recovery as this may prevent psychiatric destabilisation that could lead to relapse of the substance use disorder.

Safety

➤ Safety of the individual, family and professional are the prerequisite for any evaluation. Psychopharmacological treatments, such as antipsychotics for acute psychosis or benzodiazepines for severe alcohol withdrawal, are critical elements in any safety plan to enable individuals to establish behavioural control. The same evidence-based strategies are used for individuals experiencing combined mental health–substance use disorders as those with a single disorder.

Integrated assessment

One of the most challenging aspects of caring for individuals experiencing mental health–substance use disorders is obtaining an accurate and timely diagnosis of persistent psychiatric disorders, given the overlap of the symptoms with those of substance use disorders. Assessment and diagnosis of individuals experiencing mental health–substance use disorders is grounded in a process of **integrated, longitudinal, strength-based assessment** (ILSA) as outlined in the *Center for Substance Abuse Treatment Improvement Protocol #42.*[8] Features of the process include:

➤ Assessment begins as soon as the individual enters care, safety is assured and a history can be obtained from the individual or collateral sources.
➤ Assessment incorporates a detailed chronology of both disorders emphasising
  − onset of the substance use and psychiatric disorder
  − demonstrated history of persistent disorders
  − identification of periods of time since the onset of mental health symptoms, when the individual was not using substances, or using substances minimally, for 30 days or longer
  − careful delineation of mental illness symptoms, and responses to treatment, during those periods when substance use is at baseline, and vice versa
  − description of effects of previous treatment interventions, particularly during periods of stability
  − contributions to stability and relapse of each disorder.

KEY POINT 13.4

A thorough assessment can provide reliable indications for diagnosis and immediate initiation or continuation of psychopharmacological treatment, even for individuals who are actively using substances.

Experienced professionals recognise that many individuals need to be assessed as accurately as possible prior to their being able to achieve a 30-day period of sobriety. A careful and comprehensive integrated longitudinal assessment can provide a reliable psychiatric diagnosis and valid indications for treatment even in people who are actively using. The reliability of the diagnosis based on history argues for immediate initiation or continuation of psychopharmacological treatment (for example, antipsychotic for schizophrenia or buprenorphine for opioid maintenance). Such empirical prescribing is strongly recommended for individuals who have serious mental illness with acute symptoms. However, the converse also applies. If, after reasonable efforts to obtain a history, the diagnosis is still unclear, and the mental illness does not appear serious, attention may need to be shifted to reduction or cessation of substance use. This strategy will allow a more accurate diagnosis, even while continuing necessary interventions to safely engage the individual in continuing treatment relationships.

KEY POINT 13.5

A thorough assessment can provide reliable indications for substance use disorder and immediate initiation or continuation of psychopharmacological treatment, even for individuals who are psychiatrically destabilised.

Conversely, ILSA conducted during periods of stabilisation may provide evidence that warrants modifying or changing a previous diagnosis leading to careful discontinuation or a switch of medications because:
➤ the medication seems to have no further diagnostic indication – for example, a mood stabiliser for an individual who appeared manic when heavily using cocaine
➤ the disorder for which it was prescribed has resolved – for example, substance-induced psychosis for a person with amphetamine dependence
➤ on more extensive or longitudinal evaluation, criteria for the disorder are no longer met. (*Not all persistent disorders are permanent.*)

Continuity: initiation and maintenance of necessary medications

Non-addictive medications that are necessary for the treatment of serious mental illnesses must be initiated or maintained despite continued substance use. High-risk patterns of substance use are not a reason to discontinue medications, but indicate a need to increase monitoring and supervision. Even individuals actively using heroin who simultaneously meet historical and current criteria for a diagnosable mood or an anxiety disorder may merit pharmacological treatment with a selective SSRI.[9] Continual re-evaluation of both diagnosis and medication regimens should be the hallmark of an ongoing psychopharmacological relationship. Aims of the continuity approach to medication management are the following:
➤ to continually re-evaluate psychopharmacologic strategies to ensure the most effectively matched intervention, as the individual moves through various phases of recovery and stages of change
➤ to discontinue medication for disorders that have resolved or from which people have recovered

➤ to discontinue medications that have intolerable side effects, or have lost efficacy

➤ to cautiously taper medications for disorders where the diagnosis is no longer supported, while monitoring for recurrence or relapse of symptoms.

Expert and peer consultation for challenging situations

One of the most important resources for every prescriber is access to expert and peer consultation. Consultation is both a clinical support and a risk management strategy when faced with ethical or legal concerns. Many systems have now established formal practice guidelines for the psychopharmacologic treatment of mental health–substance use disorders, which include specific mechanisms for obtaining consultation or peer review and defined indications for which such consultation is expected.[10]

Some examples of when consultation would be strongly recommended because of the high potential risk are as follows:

➤ Continuation of treatment with benzodiazepines for an anxiety disorder beyond the period of detoxification in people with a history of substance dependence.

➤ Continuation of opioids for chronic pain in individuals who are abusing the medications, or who have known substance dependence.

➤ Discontinuation of clinically indicated medications such as antipsychotics for a person actively using substances who also has a serious persistent psychosis.

➤ Unilateral termination of treatment relationship for any individual experiencing mental health–substance use disorders.

KEY POINT 13.6

In people with psychotic disorders with or without substance use, initiation of pharmacological treatment is often urgent

---

➤ For individuals with high-risk presentations such as command homicidal ideation, there is an urgent need to establish a trusting, therapeutic alliance that will allow initiation of medications that takes priority over diagnostic certainty.

Strategies for treatment of mood and anxiety disorders

Some individuals develop substance use disorders as a form of self-medication due to inability to tolerate painful and distressing feelings or emotions.[11] To avoid reinforcing such behaviour in individuals with known substance dependence:

➤ Prescribe psychotropics to treat known or probable psychiatric disorders, not to medicate painful feelings.

➤ Advise/inform individuals that, although substances may provide short-term relief for both painful feelings and symptoms of illness, they generally create a 'rebound effect' that results in the baseline feelings or symptoms getting worse.

➤ Explain that the purpose of prescribing is not to 'take away the pain and problems of living' but to correct any 'chemical imbalance' associated with a mental illness that may lead individuals to experience their normal feelings inaccurately. Medication will thus help individuals to realistically experience, and constructively cope with, everyday emotions, even when they may be quite distressing.

➤ When medications are used to treat addictions, or psychiatric disorders, insist that medications are ancillary to a comprehensive programme:
 − the use of medication does not eliminate the need for the individual to be fully engaged to 'do the work' of recovery.

➤ Individuals in early recovery have difficulty regulating internal states and corresponding medication use; 'if some is good, more is better'. Thus, prescribers should avoid 'PRN' (*pro re nata* – as the circumstances arise) prescribing for mood and anxiety symptoms, in favour of scheduled dosing.

DIAGNOSIS-SPECIFIC PSYCHOPHARMACOLOGICAL TREATMENT FOR MENTAL ILLNESS

Best practice for treating mental illness in individuals experiencing mental health–substance use disorders is to prescribe the medication that has the soundest evidence base for the particular clinical indication notwithstanding the substance use disorders. Available research including practice guidelines and algorithms, although not specifically intended for mental health–substance use disorders, should still guide prescribing (Table 13.3). Two important exceptions are the use of benzodiazepines for anxiety disorders and opioids for chronic pain in individuals with a history of current substance dependence.

TABLE 13.3 Diagnosis-specific psychopharmacological treatment for mental illness

Disorder	Medication
Psychotic disorders	• Antipsychotics are the treatment of choice for psychosis and may improve the course of substance use disorder. • Clozapine appears to reduce substance use.[6,12] • Typical antipsychotics may be useful for acute agitation or decompensation.[13] • Typical depot antipsychotics should be considered for individuals with severe mental illness.[14] Some early evidence for depot risperidone.[15]
Bipolar disorder	• Anticonvulsants such as valproate and lamotrigine or atypical antipsychotics like olanzapine may be superior to lithium in the treatment of rapid-cycling and mixed forms of bipolar affective disorder that are more common in substance use disorders.[16,17]
Major depression	• Relative safety profile of selective serotonin reuptake inhibitors (SSRIs) and serotonin and noradrenaline reuptake inhibitors (SNRIs) gives them favourable risk/benefit over tricyclic antidepressants (TCAs) and monoamine-oxidase inhibitors (MAOIs).[18] Bupropion has a risk of seizures but may be useful for nicotine dependence in some cases.[19]

(continued)

Disorder	Medication
Major depression (*cont.*)	• SSRIs may reduce alcohol use in type II/A males with or without depression.[20]
Anxiety disorders	• Use of benzodiazepines beyond detoxification not generally warranted[21] but may be very helpful in carefully selected individuals with stable sobriety. Continuation requires consultation and risk/benefit discussion. • SSRIs, buspirone, clonidine, SNRIs are safe and effective alternatives. Atypical antipsychotics (for short-term use) and mood stabilisers such as quetiapine, gabapentin and topiramate may be useful.[22,23] • Prazosin has shown promise for post-traumatic stress disorder nightmares and flashbacks.[24]
Attention deficit hyperactivity disorder	• For both adults and adolescents, evidence is clear that if stimulants are needed to stabilise attention deficit hyperactivity disorder, they can be used safely once addiction is adequately controlled and/or the individual is properly monitored, and will be associated with better outcome for both disorders.[25–27] • Bupropion and atomoxetine are non-addictive options when the individual still is actively using or in early recovery.[26]

PSYCHOPHARMACOLOGICAL STRATEGIES IN THE TREATMENT OF SUBSTANCE USE DISORDERS

Today, there is an ever-increasing repertoire of medications listed that actually modify the craving and reward systems that underlie and drive the compulsive use that is characteristic of substance dependence (Tables 13.4, 13.5 and 13.6). **Note** that these medications are less likely to be appropriately used in individuals who only have a diagnosis of substance abuse. Preliminary evidence suggests that these agents are similarly effective in individuals with co-occurring serious mental illness.[28] This makes intuitive sense but remains an area requiring more research.

TABLE 13.4 Alcohol dependence medications

Disorder	Medication
Alcohol dependence – possibly cocaine dependence	**Disulfiram**: Interferes with metabolism of alcohol through inhibition of alcohol dehydrogenase causing an unpleasant reaction if the individual drinks. May increase psychotic symptoms necessitating increase in antipsychotic medications. Best used with cooperative or motivated individuals who are not impulsive drinkers.[29] Has been used successfully in selected individuals with serious mental illness. **Naltrexone**: An opioid antagonist shown to reduce craving for and use of alcohol by affecting reward pathways. An injectable form is also now available.[30] Has been used successfully in individuals experiencing schizophrenia. **Acamprosate**: Successfully used in Europe; results in the US have been more mixed. Reduces alcohol craving and use through glutaminergic actions.

TABLE 13.5 Medications for opioid dependence

Opioid dependence	**Methadone**: An effective form of maintenance therapy that decreases use and improves treatment retention.[31] There are recent concerns about safety including overdose and QT prolongation.[32] Multiple drug interactions and regulatory requirements complicate use.
	Naltrexone: Opioid receptor antagonist for which treatment retention is crucial to medication efficacy.[33] Has been combined successfully with positive contingencies to promote treatment adherence.
	Buprenorphine: A partial agonist used in office-based practice for certified physicians. Combined with naloxone in sublingual form to reduce diversion. Drug is easer to use, safer in overdose, less abusable and with milder withdrawal than methadone.

TABLE 13.6 Medications for cocaine dependence

Cocaine dependence	**Disulfiram**: Reduces cocaine craving and use through dopamine hydroxylase inhibition that can also worsen psychosis.[34]
	Baclofen: Preliminary indication of reduction in cocaine craving, but less robust evidence in more recent studies.[35]

COMBINED TREATMENT FOR MENTAL HEALTH–SUBSTANCE USE DISORDERS

For true and lasting recovery, medications for either mental illness or substance use must be combined with other psychosocial interventions in which the individual:

➤ receives education about the nature of mental health–substance use disorders and risks and benefits of medication

➤ participates in decision-making in a treatment partnership with the prescriber

➤ is provided stage-specific motivational enhancement therapy

➤ has access to peer support to provide information and reinforce good decisions about using substances and taking medications.

CONCLUSION

A person-centred approach that integrates evidence-based medications for the treatment of mental illness and substance use with appropriate psychosocial therapies holds the promise of improving the quality of care and the life of the individual. When confronting the complex needs and concerns of people experiencing mental health–substance use disorders, professionals will find that development of essential knowledge and skills such as outlined in this chapter will help them to provide comprehensive, effective and innovative interventions.

REFERENCES

1 Center for Substance Abuse Treatment. Substance abuse treatment for persons with co-occurring disorders. In: *Administration SAMHSA*, editor. Rockville, MD; 2005. Available at: www.ncbi.nlm.nih.gov/bookshelf/br.fcgi?book=hssamhsatip&part=A74073 (accessed 9 October 2010).

2 Minkoff K, Cline CA. Changing the world: the design and implementation of comprehensive

continuous integrated systems of care for individuals with co-occurring disorders. *Psychiatric Clinics of North America*. 2004; **27**: 727–43.

3 Montoya ID, Vocci F. Novel medications to treat addictive disorders. *Current Psychiatry Reports*. 2008; **10**: 392–8.

4 Ziedonis D, Williams JM, Smelson D. Serious mental illness and tobacco addiction: a model program to address this common but neglected issue. *American Journal of Medical Science*. 2003; **326**: 223–30.

5 Fiore MC, Bailey WC, Cohen SJ, *et al*. *Treating Tobacco Use and Dependence: a clinical practice guideline*. Rockville, MD: Public Health Service; 2000.

6 Albanese MJ, Khantzian EJ, Murphy SL, *et al*. Decreased substance use in chronically psychotic patients treated with clozapine. *American Journal of Psychiatry*. 1994; **151**: 780–1.

7 Pettinati HM, Volpicelli JR, Kranzler HR, *et al*. Sertraline treatment for alcohol dependence: interactive effects of medication and alcoholic subtype. *Alcohol: Clinical and Experimental Research*. 2000; **24**: 1041–9.

8 Center for Substance Abuse Treatment. *Substance Abuse Treatment for Persons With Co-occurring Disorders*. Treatment Improvement Protocol (TIP) Series 42. DHHS Publication No. (SMA) 05–3922. Rockville, MD: Substance Abuse and Mental Health Services Administration; 2005.

9 Stein MD, Solomon DA, Anderson BJ, *et al*. Persistence of antidepressant treatment effects in a pharmacotherapy plus psychotherapy trial for active injection drug users. *American Journal of Addiction*. 2005; **14**: 346–57.

10 Minkoff K. *Comprehensive Continuous Integrated System of Care (CCICS): psychopharmacology practice guideline for individuals with co-occurring psychiatric and substance use disorders (COD)*. Harvard, MA; 2005. Available at: www.bhrm.org/guidelines/ddguidelines. htm (accessed 9 October 2010).

11 Bizzarri JV, Rucci P, Sbrana A, *et al*. Substance use in severe mental illness: self-medication and vulnerability factors. *Psychiatry Research*. 2009; **165**: 88–95.

12 Zimmet SV, Strous RD, Burgess ES, *et al*. Effects of clozapine on substance use in patients with schizophrenia and schizoaffective disorder: a retrospective survey. *Journal of Clinical Psychopharmacology*. 2000; **20**: 94–8.

13 Allen MH, Currier GW, Hughes DH, *et al*. Treatment of behavioral emergencies: a summary of the expert consensus guidelines. *Journal of Psychiatric Practice*. 2003; **9**: 16–38.

14 Shi L, Ascher-Svanum H, Zhu B, *et al*. Characteristics and use patterns of patients taking first-generation depot antipsychotics or oral antipsychotics for schizophrenia. *Psychiatric Services*. 2007; **58**: 482–8.

15 Rubio G, Martinez I, Ponce G, *et al*. Long-acting injectable risperidone compared with zuclopenthixol in the treatment of schizophrenia with substance abuse comorbidity. *Canadian Journal of Psychiatry*. 2006; **51**: 531–9.

16 Ostacher MJ, Sachs GS. Update on bipolar disorder and substance abuse: recent findings and treatment strategies. *Journal of Clinical Psychiatry*. 2006; **67**: e10.

17 Goldberg JF. Bipolar disorder with comorbid substance abuse: diagnosis, prognosis, and treatment. *Journal of Psychiatric Practice*. 2001; **7**: 109–22.

18 American Psychiatric Association. *Practice Guideline for the Treatment of Substance Use Disorders*. American Psychiatric Association Practice Guidelines for the Treatment of Psychiatric Disorders: Compendium 2006. 2nd ed. Arlington, VA: American Psychiatric Association; 2006. pp. 291–563.

19 Zwar N, Richmond R. Bupropion sustained release: a therapeutic review of Zyban. *Australian Family Physician*. 2002; **31**: 443–7.

20 Pettinati HM, Dundon W, Lipkin C. Gender differences in response to sertraline pharmacotherapy in Type A alcohol dependence. *American Journal of Addiction*. 2004; **13**: 236–47.

21 Ciraulo DA, Nace EP. Benzodiazepine treatment of anxiety or insomnia in substance abuse patients. *American Journal of Addiction*. 2000; **9**: 276–9; discussion pp. 280–4.

22 Sowers W, Golden S. Psychotropic medication management in persons with co-occurring psychiatric and substance use disorders. *Journal of Psychoactive Drugs*. 1999; **31**: 59–70.

23 Myrick H, Brady K. Current review of the comorbidity of affective, anxiety, and substance use disorders. *Current Opinion in Psychiatry*. 2003; **16**: 261–70.

24 Taylor FB, Martin P, Thompson C, *et al*. Prazosin effects on objective sleep measures and clinical symptoms in civilian trauma posttraumatic stress disorder: a placebo-controlled study. *Biological Psychiatry*. 2008; **63**: 629–32.

25 Biederman J, Wilens T, Mick E, *et al*. Pharmacotherapy of attention-deficit/hyperactivity disorder reduces risk for substance use disorder. *Pediatrics*. 1999; **104**: e20.

26 Kollins SH. A qualitative review of issues arising in the use of psycho-stimulant medications in patients with ADHD and co-morbid substance use disorders. *Current Medical Research and Opinion*. 2008; **24**: 1345–57.

27 Peterson K, McDonagh MS, Fu R. Comparative benefits and harms of competing medications for adults with attention-deficit hyperactivity disorder: a systematic review and indirect comparison meta-analysis. *Psychopharmacology (Berlin)*. 2008; **197**: 1–11.

28 Batki SL, Dimmock JA, Wade M, *et al*. Monitored naltrexone without counseling for alcohol abuse/dependence in schizophrenia-spectrum disorders. *American Journal of Addiction*. 2007; **16**: 253–9.

29 Mueser KT, Noordsy DL, Fox L, *et al*. Disulfiram treatment for alcoholism in severe mental illness. *American Journal of Addiction*. 2003; **12**: 242–52.

30 Garbutt JC, Kranzler HR, O'Malley SS, *et al*. Efficacy and tolerability of long-acting injectable naltrexone for alcohol dependence: a randomized controlled trial. *Journal of the American Medical Association*. 2005; **293**: 1617–25.

31 Mattick RP, Breen C, Kimber J, *et al*. Methadone maintenance therapy versus no opioid replacement therapy for opioid dependence. *Cochrane Database Syst Rev*. 2009 Jul 8; (3):CD002209.

32 Krantz MJ, Martin J, Stimmel B, *et al*. QTc interval screening in methadone treatment. *Annals Internal Medicine*. 2009; **150**: 387–95.

33 Johansson BA, Berglund M, Lindgren A. Efficacy of maintenance treatment with naltrexone for opioid dependence: a meta-analytical review. *Addiction*. 2006; **101**: 491–503.

34 Carroll KM, Fenton LR, Ball SA, *et al*. Efficacy of disulfiram and cognitive behavior therapy in cocaine-dependent outpatients: a randomized placebo-controlled trial. *Archives of General Psychiatry*. 2004; **61**: 264–72.

35 Haney M, Hart CL, Foltin RW. Effects of baclofen on cocaine self-administration: opioid- and nonopioid-dependent volunteers. *Neuropsychopharmacology*. 2006; **31**: 1814–21.

TO LEARN MORE

- American Psychiatric Association Steering Committee on Practice Guidelines. Treatment of patients with substance use disorders, 2nd ed. *American Journal of Psychiatry*. 2007; **164** (4 Suppl.): 5–123.
- Geppert C, Minkoff K. *Psychiatric Disorders and Medications*. Center City, MN: Hazelden; 2003.
- Geppert C, Minkoff K. *Psychiatric Medications and Recovery from Co-occurring Disorders*. Center City, MN: Hazelden; 2003.

- Center for Substance Abuse Treatment. *Substance Abuse Treatment for Persons with Co-occurring Disorders: treatment improvement protocol #42*, CSAT, Washington: 2005. Available at: www.ncbi.nlm.nih.gov/bookshelf/br.fcgi?book=hssamhsatip&part=A74073 (accessed 23 January 2011).

CHAPTER 14

Complementary and alternative therapies: magic, mystery or fact?

Je Kan Adler-Collins

INTRODUCTION

I was working in a Buddhist hospice in north-west Thailand when, with considerable surprise, I opened an email inviting me to contribute a section in what appears to be a selection of books written by mental healthcare professionals, of which I am definitely not one. I was so certain that it was a mistake, and they must be thinking of someone else, that I checked and rechecked with the editor. It appears that no mistake has been made, and I am excited to offer insights to what I do in my work in relation to mental wholeness and well-being. However, before I start, I have to make the space safe for my reader, as I understand that the written word is never the received word and as a Buddhist monk I believe that I have to make transparent my values in order to defuse the possible misunderstandings that can occur when a reader engages with a text that comes from a different sense of being and culture.

As a Western (British) nurse and professional educator I am aware that academic writing is often expected in such texts as this. I also checked on this as I have no wish to place my words and work in an exclusive frame of academic writing, formatting and reference. I have enough issues with this in writing for nursing journals, which is a requirement of an academic position. I believe I have good reason for not wanting to do this as most of my references and learning come from texts that are thousands of years old via translations, oral histories, folk history, healing dances, circles and ceremonies. It is a uniquely Western mannerism to assume that you own knowledge or your name should be attributed to certain texts, values and ideas. History is full of some very famous people having their names linked to certain texts and discoveries. Modern research and the application of rigorous cross-referencing and indexing via global networks of scholars is revealing that much of what was discovered by the West had been discovered many thousands of years before in China, for example, but is still incorrectly attributed in even modern reference texts. This knowledge was not owned by any one individual and as such this text is my representation of my knowing and understandings, which have been informed by countless thousands of others. Therefore, I am not its owner but the dubious guardian of a very fluid state of understanding as consciousness fluctuates from question to question, informed by what I see in my practice and my travels.

SELF-ASSESSMENT EXERCISE 14.1

> **Time: 20 minutes**
> Consider your own breadth and depth of 'knowledge'. Where does it come from? Think in broad terms.

I choose to narrate my story of my learning and engagement with complementary and alternative therapies through the windows of my practice. I wish to tell how my knowing evolved through trial and error combined with the necessity of circumstances. I am aware that a complex set of issues surrounds the use of complementary medicine in the West, and various bodies lay claim to its ownership. Many in positions of power seek to discredit its use or place it into a bio-medical model of efficacy and evidence while at the same time excluding spirituality and mystery as part of our basic human heritage. This text is not the place for that debate as what I write is closely linked to my values as a Buddhist monk and the research that I have carried out over the past decade into alternative therapies in Asia. Even the use of the word 'alternative' is a Western term coined by the medical and new-age lobbies. In many parts of the world natural medicine is the norm not the alternative.

SELF-ASSESSMENT EXERCISE 14.2

> **Time: 20 minutes**
> If 'alternative' means the possibility of choice, what realistic choices are offered for people experiencing mental health–substance use concerns and dilemmas in terms of alternative therapies?

In this text, I actively question my understanding of what mental health is and how it is managed. I seriously question the ongoing fragmentation of knowing and knowledge into ever-decreasing bits of expertise. I fully acknowledge that some will feel that I have gone native so to speak, and having passed through the United Kingdom education system and being awarded my PhD in education in 2007, I have come to realise that Western forms of education actively bring about a sense of separation and a focus on the individual self as the norm for our humanness. It is this sense of separation that allows us not to practise integrated wholeness of healthcare. Understanding this concept set my course of action as I questioned the peddling of concepts of healthcare alongside the global industrial might of wealth care. I seek answers to why we have such ever-increasing manifestation of disease and hold the understanding that most suffering is a result of dis-ease, a form of discontent that brings about spiritual, physical, mental and emotional distress. I acknowledge that there is a place for medication in the treatment of disease but question the overprescription of mind- or state-altering medication and the dependency it can so easily produce. These ideas are discussed in the text as they emerged from the people I care for.

WHAT THIS TEXT IS AND IS NOT

As already stated this text is a story of exploration and understanding grounded in the delivery of care to people suffering with mental dis-ease through the medium of integrated care. It is not a reference work on complementary therapies or mental health conditions nor should it be approached as one. Care should be taken not to take the ideas and methods out of context as they could cause further dis-ease. Extensive training of esoteric healing methods and concepts is needed to practise these techniques and should not be attempted by the layperson. What is written in this text does not replace the advice of a mental health professional.

UNDERPINNING ONTOLOGY

I am a Buddhist monk of Shingon Shu esoteric Buddhism in Japan. I find it a disciplined and challenging form of Buddhism that supports my enquiry into my lifelong learning and the growth of my understanding as I reconnect to the elements in a journey of my healing of my mental wellness. Part of this understanding is that our consciousness attends the University of Physical Life in order to see our humanness as it really is. Our world as we understand it is a matrix of impulses and data provided by our senses. Each of us lives in a world of one, created by us for us. No one else can see or feel or construct our world. In that sense, we are unique and original. Buddhism suggests that all forms of consciousness are linked to the mental body or described as mental causation. We attach ourselves to this as a form of certainty. The form of certainty is attributed to our sense of everyday-ness or repeatability. This in turn, through its repetition, creates pathways of assumed knowing. As this text is not an engagement with Buddhism in its many forms, I shall only refer to concepts that can assist the reader to see how the flow of logic is applied to the process of dis-ease as I understand it.

SELF-ASSESSMENT EXERCISE 14.3

Time: 20 minutes
Consider the concept of 'suffering'. What feelings arise in you when you feel helpless to prevent suffering in others?

THE CONCEPT OF SUFFERING

Within all actions, feelings and emotions there exists the potential for the opposite. One of the core concepts for a Buddhist monk is to help in the relief of suffering in others. So, for example, the pursuit of happiness has within it the seeds of unhappiness. Holding on to the illusion of happiness causes us to struggle when we lose that state and move into unhappiness. A more useful approach is to focus on the middle way, neither happy nor sad but allowing all circumstances to reveal their teachings to you. Such an approach uses meditation in its varying forms to reflect and enquire of just how the matrix of selfhood has been constructed. This mindful approach to existence sees opportunities for learning and the deepening of understanding in the everyday moments of life. It also explores the concepts of time and space, one where the ideas of our humanness are part of an integrated concept of creation, a fusion of spiritual, mental, emotional, physical and environmental conditioning and integrated matrices of understanding.

THE CONCEPT OF COMPASSION

It is my understanding and belief that compassion is a state of loving acceptance in a universal sense. I see the suffering in the individual and seek to bring them to their own understanding of how and why they are suffering. Compassion does not judge the individual nor does it suggest that the consequences of an action will not be painful to those whom experience them. Compassion sees all actions as choices made to bring about learning and enlightenment. Compassion does not condone violence as a solution but seeks to create safe spaces for healing and understanding. Sometimes holding compassion as a lived value appears to be like trying to hold the world on your shoulders and so often your heart just wants to break – and sometimes it does. I believe compassion is a form of love, a belief in the potential for good in people, although sometimes you have to look very hard to find it.

CONCEPTUALISING SPACE

Eastern teachings tell us that we are created from the elements; some teach four:
1 earth
2 water
3 fire
4 wind.

Some include a fifth such as wood or cosmos. Each element is a force within itself or an elemental and each element has properties attributed. Disease is essentially when the space occupied by our biological mass (physical body) experiences a dis-harmony with either the inner space (inside the body) or outer space (environmental and social context). The interphases between inner and outer spaces are the emotional body and the mental body. The glue, as it were, for keeping all these different aspects of selfhood in some sort of functional order, is that of spirituality, which flows like a life force among all states of being.

Space is an important concept to my understanding, as we all share the same space. By this, I mean that to date nothing solid has been found in this creation by our hard-working scientists. What has been found are different holes in space that lead to other spaces. Buddhists believe that forms create space so the biological form of the mass of your body creates a space for itself in space (cellular division) and time (biological clocks). In this sense, we, and everything in the creation, are connected in the same space.

The Western concept of a distinct and separate self is perhaps the root cause for most forms of dis-ease. To see one's self as an individual immediately fragments that individual from the collective whole. A sense of dis-ease and disconnectedness takes root in our consciousness. The flow of life-affirming energy is known by many names in different cultures: the toa, chi, ki, life force, universal energy, spirit, to name but a few. This sense of separation and loss of identification or/and connection to the environment and elements makes it easy for us to be totally destructive, for if we have no connection to water, for example, it is easy to pollute it, and if we lose our connection to nature, then it is easy to destroy it in the hopeless task of sustaining an illusionary state of self.

The essence of my work is seeking ways to bring about a reintegration of the assumed self with its self-destructive focus on its own wants and needs, to a more-integrated understanding of our unique place in the order of things, and a closer understanding of the beauty we share with our environment and the elements. This may seem highly esoteric and completely impractical so I will use a sample case study as an exemplar of how a positive outcome from this approach can be achieved. This is not being offered as a model in the Western sense but rather as a window into a new approach to integrated healthcare, which may or may not have relevance to your working situation.

A very wise person once said that our body is a house with many rooms. I believe that each of our bodies, Spiritual, Mental, Emotional and Physical, are houses in a neighbourhood of selfhood. Each is linked to the other by many doors. Parts of this neighbourhood we know very well and we gain a sense of comfort from our knowingness. Parts we do not know or have not explored and, thus, these remain closed and potentially fearful. Others we have touched lightly and found we do not like the space, so we lock the doors hoping never to return. We each create pathways of reliability between our different houses. Reliable in the sense that we have trodden them often and can easily navigate our way to whatever room in whatever house our consciousness wishes to place itself. When these pathways become blocked or closed, the flow of energy diverts or builds up and opens doors into new, unexplored parts of our houses. The matrix of our reality can no longer sustain itself and the old, familiar pathways are gone. This leads to a breaking down of old patterning and, as we shall see from the case study, this breaking down can be a very positive experience when approached with a non-judgemental mindset. In the event of such a point being reached for whatever reason, I believe that we pass through three distinct stages of a process, each of which requires slightly differing approaches to facilitate recovery.

1 The casualty stage

Bad things happen to good people, and we never know when a trauma is going to present itself to us or if the unique set of coping mechanisms we have developed will cope. The casualty stage is one where we cannot cope with what is or has happened. It does not mean that we are weak-willed or lack moral fibre, or that we are bad people. It is a simple statement of fact. If you have broken your leg, you cannot walk. If part of your thinking process breaks, you cannot think, or you think in a very strange manner. Becoming a casualty is from a Buddhist perspective a great opportunity for learning. We have to face complex issues of dependence on others, vulnerability, trusting others to care for us, loss of individual power and status, helplessness, pain, grief or/and perhaps a loss. All of these have both negative and positive aspects to them. What is interesting about these situations is they usually occur as a result of the existing coping system or patterning not working, so the mind is making a new map under pressure so to speak, and usually the most dominant emotions and feelings are negative. Thus, the mind creates a new room where the doors have been forced open among the different neighbourhoods of self. The flow of life energy or Ki is no longer smooth but disrupted or even blocked, and in some cases it just flows in circular patterns like a whirlpool going nowhere. The casualty stage has its phases:

➤ event or trauma
➤ acceptance or denial
➤ recovery
➤ victim.

We experience each of these stages in the growth of our understanding of the human experience.

2 The survivor stage

This stage is one where the body recognises that it is in trouble or is experiencing stress but, because of personality, training (as in the military, first responders or emergency services), these individuals quickly rise to the situation and are often efficient organisers in a crisis. However, in the survivor, these are suppressed, and they function on existing patterning and training. I believe, however, they too are being forced into a new room, but they shut down emotionally, spirituality and mentally in order to survive and get the job done. The problem with the survivor stage is that it is setting the stage for a complex conditioning where I believe more than one reality can exist. The reality of the trauma is seared on the consciousness and then kept locked as the individual tries to live by another, 'normal' reality. However, the mind knows that there is unfinished business and that the shock of the trauma has not been processed. It, therefore, creates slipways in the mind where doors can open back into the trauma outside the survivor's control. If these are not treated the survivor is, in fact, a casualty; albeit not at the point of trauma, they are just as disabled.

3 The sage stage

I often imagine that the sage individual will have a sweatshirt that proclaims: been there, seen it, done it, got the video, book and film rights! – as this is what the sage has done. They have transcended through understanding, not through theory but through lived experience. The sage can recognise the patterns of casualty and survivor and speak with the street language of experience. The sage can offer advice and a map to find the individual's own way back to themself. The sage understands the self-loathing, self-deceit and self-illusion but sees the potential for good and bad in everything with infinite compassion.

These three stages do not necessarily follow one another. You may, for example, physically be a casualty, mentally be a survivor, and spiritually be a sage all at the same time, or combinations thereof, which make life interesting. You can also be stuck in casualty or survivor modes of thinking, which makes achieving states of sage-hood a challenge.

TOOLS OF BUDDHIST MINDFULNESS

At this point, I wish to clarify certain terms that will be used in the case study in order for the reader to have insights to what is embedded in the term and its function.

Breath

Breathing is our basic tool, for without breath there is no life as we understand it. Good breathing rhythms and a focus on breath help clarify the mind and bring essential oxygen to the body. An excited or agitated mind is reflected in our breathing. A focus on how we breathe and the depth of our breathing can, after practice, reduce resting breathing to four breaths a minute. This deep breathing does not cause hypoxia and an adept of breathing can go for even longer periods during deep meditation.

Meditation

Meditation is so simple and so complex, a sort of living contradiction. It has many shapes and forms, and usually you have to find the form that suits yourself. The more you seek it the more elusive it seems to become. However, the moment you stop seeking it just appears. We teach mindfulness meditation, which is to bring the focus of your mind completely into the moment to be aware or seek awareness of all that is in and around you. In our temple, you can be chopping wood or carrying water, sweeping leaves, cooking or healing. Meditation is a living state of consciousness not just limited to formal acts of reflected thinking but a natural flow of peace and harmony in your daily living. We use creative visualisation; semi-structured and structured meditations, alongside formal sitting, depending on the needs of the person.

Prayer

Prayer can mean many things to many people. For some it is everything, for others it has no function or meaning. For me, prayer is an active meditation where chanting Sanskrit and specific hand movements are used to engage the chatterbox of chaos in the mind, and after several hundred repetitions the frequency of the prayer brings about certain insights. Buddhists do not believe in the concept of a divine God deity, sitting in judgement or able to intervene in the ways and actions of humankind. Our prayers are directed to the Buddha (Teacher) that we believe is inside us and when awakened can teach us to see ourselves and our universe as it really is and allow us to serve others with compassion.

SELF-ASSESSMENT EXERCISE 14.4

Time: 20 minutes

Think about a time when you or a family member have suffered and have been searching for answers. What/who has helped you? What do you think about the answers being within yourself? Reflect on this.

COMPLEMENTARY AND ALTERNATIVE MEDICINE

As already suggested, the very terms 'complementary' and 'alternative' medicine are highly problematic. In the United Kingdom, complementary medicine is a therapy under the care and control of a medical doctor. Alternative medicine is a course of treatment not under the control of a medical doctor but of a suitably qualified practitioner. I hardly ever use these terms now as they are attached to entrenched views of power, politics and money. I tend to use the term 'integrated care' – integrated in the sense that many disciplines are included, case by case, for the best support of the person's healing process. Wherever possible, I prefer to work with medical professionals as part of the care team, actively seeking to build up networks globally with scientists, doctors, nurses, therapists and of course individuals using the service.

INTEGRATED HEALTHCARE TOOLS: VIBRATIONAL TOOLS AND THERAPIES

Given the understanding that we are vibrational beings, and that we vibrate beyond a subatomic level, the biological mass that creates our physical bodies vibrates alongside that of all matter and mass in this universe. Even our minds have a vibration; for example, positive thinking can impact tremendously on recovery whereas negative thinking has the opposite effect. The essence of vibrational healing is to bring back the harmony and flow of life force (Chi/Ki) into the body mass. The main players in this system are those of the Hindu understanding of chakras (wheels). These energetic wheels are how the life force that is part of the flow of creation is the focus in our biological form. They could be seen as power stations, and the system of meridian lines of Chinese traditional medicine as the power grid with tsubo points (pressure points) as the substations or access points to the grid. Each wheel is given a set of values and a colour, each meridian line links to a system of the body and each tsubo gives access to open an energy point or to close one. The whole concept is about vibrational harmony with the environment and the cosmos.

Following are listed some of the main tools I use alongside a short description.

Crystal and crystal essences

Crystals have a natural beauty. They also have a very useful quality of being stable in terms of their frequency, which varies according to their chemical composition. They are useful in meditation. Crystal essences have a value attributed to them and are used to assist the person in processing an emotion or issue. I believe that they are nature's energetic surgeons and get straight to the point of dis-ease.

Flower essence and tinctures

These are a sort of cross between pure vibrational essence (homeopathy) and herbs (boiling method). They are given a set of values and taken by the individual as part of a meditation. They are surprisingly accurate in isolating the emotional issues the individual is facing. The flower essences are taken to assist processing and allow a gentle healing from the bottom up. We make them in our temple using spring water and flowering herbs. They are very gentle in their action and work well with combinations of crystal essences.

Traditional Chinese nursing

Cupping the acupuncture points is a Chinese technique for releasing blockages and encouraging the flow of Chi around the body. Burning Chinese herbs can be applied in massage to specific acupuncture points. Massage with herbal preparations using cupping or a wooden/bone spatula stimulates circulation and detoxification of the physical body.

Massage and body work

I use many types of massage with oils, herbs or aromatherapy essential oils. Massage is still one of the best ways to remove tension and re-programme the body through positive touch.

Thai herbs, applied topically by hot massage or steam baths and sauna, are also taken in the detoxification phase at the start of the treatment.

Waterfall meditation

In Japanese this is called Mizugyo (water test). It involves entering a natural spring pool that has a waterfall and meditating, at first in the pool and then in the waterfall. It is hard to explain how it works but the cold water and the meditation have a grounding effect on the body. It discharges the mind so to speak as the falling water hits the head almost like a repolarisation of the brain. The cold takes your breath away, and you have to focus on the body's natural responses to cold water. However, against the odds you soon start to feel warm and refreshed. It is a great place for discharging anger or sorrow. It remains one of the great mysteries why this treatment is so effective.

Sweat lodge

Used for centuries by many different cultures, the mindful building of the sweat lodge with its associated spiritual and healing connections provides a good space for detoxification, sharing and storytelling. The main problem is having gatekeepers and especially a fire keeper with the necessary understandings and wisdom to fulfil their roles in the ceremony safely.

Philosophy of care

Underpinning all our approaches to caring is the central theme of the relief of suffering. If the individual is suffering then so are we, for such individuals are an integral part of our community when they are in our care. By this, I mean the whole community supports the healing process for we believe that the dis-ease being experienced and being expressed by the individual is but a reflection of our own. So, for example, if the individual has to do water meditation we all do water meditation with them. We are not into long, convoluted therapy sessions where all aspects of an individual's life are discussed, but of course we offer counselling support. We do this by creating spaces for listening. We observe the individual's actions and use silence as a medium of communication. We allow nature to do the healing with the flower essences supporting body work and, finally, outside physical work. Because we believe that separation is a prime cause for most dis-ease we encourage the individual to fill their time with periods of constructive work and planned

rests. If the individual would like to take a bath, no problems; they just have to collect the wood, chop the wood and light the fire to the outside bath. Through this
experience – the fact that producing hot water requires a lot of effort, planning and
new skill sets – the individuals begin to learn how conditioned they have become
to immediacy of utilities, food and services. We grow a lot of our own food and
this requires considerable effort to maintain the gardens and fruit trees. Chickens
produce our eggs and require a lot of care. All work tasks are essential parts of our
community life. No task is given just for its own sake and individuals can soon see
the results of their work. Cooking, baking, preserving, washing, cleaning is all part
of normal life, and the individual is expected to do her/his share of the work. We
start with small, easily achieved tasks slowly building up to the person accepting
more responsibility for the community as their programme progresses.

Entry into our care is voluntary. We have no restraining policy and people can
leave whenever they wish. The fact we are located on the top of a mountain in a
forest 30 minutes away by car from the nearest small rural shop means that considerable effort is needed to find us and get to us. Absconding has not been an issue,
strangely, nor has incompletion of their healing programme. Family members can
stay in alternative accommodation at the temple. However, we usually like there to
be a period of no physical contact with family and friends as the first month of the
programme is usually a detoxification period. This can be quite a difficult time as
people arrive in varying degrees of toxicity and distress. Often just the silence of the
space can be an issue for an individual who has filled their life with noise, television,
radio, pop videos or work. There is no mobile phone contact on our mountain,
no televisions, no radios, no traffic noise or the hustle and bustle of a city. Noise
withdrawal can be a big issue to deal with. We do have ADSL Internet, and Skype
communications are a useful way to keep families informed. We usually request that
all medications be stopped before the stay, where medically possible – insulin for
diabetes, for example, would not be stopped. No non-essential medications, sleeping tablets, psychiatric medications such as Prozac or diazepam, diet supplements
and so forth are taken away. The dosage and amount of time the individual has been
taking their medication can drastically alter how the programme is planned. Our
next step is a very clear informed consent and waiver document, which is signed
by the individual, if over the age of consent, and the family (not always possible as
some families are estranged). Some people come as private individuals, as privacy
and confidentiality are major aspects of our care.

AN EXAMPLE

A 23-year-old former model turned TV entertainer/singer.

Clinical diagnosis (medical) 'eating disorder' . . . anorexia with bulimia.
Depressive episodes.

This young woman presented with a history of dieting as a professional model
from the age of 13 and as her career became more successful she moved into
television drama and singing. The dieting became compulsive, compounded with
bulimia. She had a long history of taking diet pills, combined with stimulants, and
admitted mild usage of recreational drugs, the main ones being cocaine, and

ecstasy. She was beautifully dressed in fashionable oversized clothes, wore semi-opaque sunglasses, and her hair was covered by a baseball cap. As with all new people, we ask them to take a bath and change into the temple working clothes that we all wear. Further discussion and care planning would take place after she had settled into her sleeping space, which she shares with other temple staff (nuns and temple volunteers). We do this so that all makeup and professional hair crafting has been removed and the individual's body is in its natural state. It is the only time during her initial stay where she has the bath made for her.

The second interview presented a very different picture, that of a very sick and pale woman. Her eyes were sunken and mirrored by dark rings (a sign of spleen chi deficiency). Her eyes were filled with shame and despair plus a degree of hopelessness. Her skin was pale and dry with poor elasticity response. Hair was dry and limp with a slight crackly feel to it. The ends were split. Oral hygiene was good but her breath smelt of ketosis and her gums bled easily. She looked anaemic with pale inner eyelids. Her nails were ridged and she had a slight hand tremor. Chest was clear, but abdomen presented with painful liver, stomach and gut. Her hydration was good and her urine output satisfactory. She had been having irregular menstruation for the last few years and was uncertain when the next one was due. Her bowel movements were problematic due to her frequent use of laxatives and enemas, and she alternated between constipation and diarrhoea. Her loss of body mass and muscle tone was extensive with a body weight of 42 kg and a height of 155 cm.

After a full medical case history had been taken, informed consent was obtained, which has greater importance in this case as she would be on 24-hour watch. This means that she is escorted to the toilet if she needs to use the toilet within four hours of eating. Self-induced vomiting is a form of violence to your own body. Our policy is zero tolerance to violence of any sort, and to prevent this, a close watch is kept on the individual.

The next stage of the process is detoxification. This usually entails taking a selection of Thai herbs at 4.30 in the morning and the system is usually cleansed by midday. This was not an option in this case due to the issues with her bowels and the fragility of her condition. It was decided that any therapy or intervention that could cause further trauma to the body could be placed on hold until she was stronger. Her process for the next few weeks became just plain old tender love and care. She was massaged twice a day with warm oils, participated in meditations and helped with light tasks around the temple. She was also supported by the flower essences, one of which is California poppy. This is the unsung hero of addictive behaviour patterning. No special issue was made of her problems with food; she was given small portions of organic, wholesome Japanese vegetarian food with the rest of the temple at meal times, supplemented by fresh fruits, nuts and high-fibre dried fruits. Soya milk was used instead of dairy milk and cheeses were used sparingly in her diet at first. At no point was she asked to talk about her condition. It was for her to instigate any conversations relating to herself. Slowly, over time, bits of her history and the underlying issues started to surface. She was a child star after being entered in a local photo contest at 11 years of age. Her parents dominated her training in music, dance, deportment and pageant politics.

She was never allowed to have friends or get her nails broken. She could not play games with her friends in case of an injury that would cancel a photo shoot. Her world consisted of different groups of people who were manipulating her for their own needs, usually for profit. She felt like a packaged piece of property and somewhere in the process she lost her identity of who she was. She soon learned from other girls that a way to exercise some form of control and get back a small amount of personal power was to use her body as a weapon against those whom she felt were using her. In her own words she said 'I just wanted it to stop but did not know how. I was on a glitzy roller coaster of fame fortune and excitement; there was no way off, no one would listen. If I became ugly no one would want me, and it would all be OK'. Once the inner issues had surfaced it was just a matter of supporting her as she reviewed her feelings about them. After three weeks, she was strong enough to do detoxification, which proceeded with no mishaps, and she then started doing Mizugyo, where she processed a lot of her anger.

We have a simple philosophy when dealing with issues around biological parents and that is, no matter what they did or did not do, they gave you the gift of life. For this, each day in your prayers, you should give thanks because without them you would not exist. Understanding this has a powerful healing property and in many cases allows for the first stage of forgiveness to start its healing process. We also work with the concept of the karmic law of return; this means that in your many incarnations the good actions and the bad actions have to balance out. Everything in our lives is as it should be. It is a tough call living with such an understanding. Accepting responsibility for what happens in your life as a potential learning experience – which can facilitate the practice of compassion and spiritual growth – will often give the person the chance to step outside the frame of his/her own thinking and seek to understand the thinking of those whom they perceived to have hurt them. It is often the case that when examined from a different perspective, sometimes the actions of others (who were doing their best – as they thought – given their life circumstances and context), can actually reveal how much they gave in their own way and this can facilitate the process of forgiveness. Sometimes, however, no matter how hard you look, you cannot find the good, and then in such circumstances you are learning about unconditional forgiveness. This, at times, seems impossible as we scream out for revenge, for justice to be seen to be done. We demand some form of payment, retribution for our pain. The answer to injustice is not justice but unconditional love, starting with yourself.

Slowly, but steadily she gained body mass from a well-balanced diet and working outdoors. The next stage of her recovery was assisting her to realise that the old understanding of her self-identity and lifestyle was unsustainable, and she needed to reflect on what she wished to do to give her life a focus and purpose. There were no easy answers to give, as it is a highly personal process. There was unfinished business in her life that needed resolution that only she could bring about. She left us after about three months when she felt she was ready. Her contacts were regular and confident at first and then soon trailed away to the occasional postcard and then nothing.

As often is the case after recovery, people do not keep in touch as we remind them of dark times in a dark space. I pray that no news is good news, and that she found the strength and the answers she needed to live her way.

HUMANNESS AND UNDERSTANDING

This case history sets the framework for our approach to anorexia, addiction and depression, which we have used on several occasions. Each case has a different underlying cause. The main difference in treatment approaches is the use of flower essences, crystal essence and herbal preparations, which changes with each individual. The number of times that each therapy is used depends on the needs of the individual. Detoxification appears to be the key to treatments. Detoxification is applicable to all the holistic bodies – spiritual, mental, emotional and physical –secure in a safe environment that is closely linked with nature – open spaces, forests, water and fresh air – and with physical work that has a visible outcome, such as gardening for growing their food, cleaning as a social community duty (e.g. toilets, public space, private space). The cleansing uses methods that reconnect to the elements as already described. However, there often comes a time when all the treatment approaches are seen for what they truly are – tools that open opportunities to communicate. In the final analysis, the individual and healthcare professional have to meet each other in the essence of their humanness. Perhaps it is this understanding that offers the most hope. In my recent research, I looked at easing distress of all the bodies in poor and socially deprived people dying from varying types of cancers. Using what we understood from our practice suggested that an integrated approach using spiritual exercises such as meditation could decrease distress, suffering and mental anguish. We used a recognised mental health instrument, culturally modified, and the measurement of stress indicators in the saliva. Both the mental health tool and the saliva tests showed marked positive responses to meditation being used as an agent to relieve mental distress.

CONCLUSION

I believe that integrated healthcare offers a set of tools to open spaces for listening to the issues of others and provides a framework for the specific needs of the individual. As part of planned strategy to wellness, integrated healthcare can offer new ways of decreasing dependency on the system to provide all the answers, and increasing personal responsibility for the individual to manage their own healthcare. I hope that this chapter has provided some ideas and new thinking about other options that exist. I wish to express my thanks to the editor in having the courage and foresight to include an offering with a different slant to mental well-being. Should you wish further communications, and I hope you do, please use the contact details provided.

CHAPTER 15

Pain management

*Peter Athanasos, Rose Neild, Charlotte de Crespigny
and Lynette Cusack*

INTRODUCTION

Pain management in the general population

One of the biggest challenges facing health professionals is adequate pain management. It is generally accepted that severe pain is poorly treated in the general population. There may be a number of reasons for this.

➤ Professionals may not prescribe adequate amounts of opioids for fear of respiratory depression or cognitive and psychomotor effects – for example, driving a car or operating machinery.

➤ The prescriber may fear the development of iatrogenic dependence – that is, causing the person to become addicted by prescribing opioids for pain. (This is a relatively rare occurrence.)

➤ The prescriber may fear that the person will divert their prescription opioid drugs if given too liberally or in excess of requirement.[1]

➤ The prescriber may also have a poor understanding of the pharmacodynamics and pharmacokinetics of medication in the context of pain and prescribe ineffectively.[2]

Pain management in the opioid-maintained population

People maintained on opioids, both for the treatment of opioid dependence (addiction) and for the treatment of chronic pain, who present to clinics and general wards with acute pain conditions are a particular challenge.[3] They may present with any of the various medical or surgical problems causing acute pain including serious illnesses, injuries and infectious diseases (e.g. hepatitis or human immunodeficiency virus – HIV). For these people acute pain management following surgery or trauma may be especially problematic. In general, the individuals experience a greater sensitivity to pain and a cross-tolerance to analgesic effects of opioids as a result of their opioid dependence. This complicates treatment considerably.

There are three complications to pain management in this population.

1 **Misunderstandings** regarding the management of acute and chronic pain.

2 **Opioid tolerance**: with opioid use, opioid tolerance develops and people require more drug to maintain the same effect.

215

3 **Hyperalgesia**: with opioid use, there may be the paradoxical development of greater pain sensitivity.[4]

Common misconceptions

Many misconceptions arise around pain management and opioid dependence due to common stereotypes associated with dependence. This stereotyping can lead to inappropriate or suboptimal pain management. For example, it is important to consider that physical dependence and tolerance are typical and predictable consequences of regular frequent opioid exposure. People who use opioids for chronic pain management or treatment of opioid dependence often become tolerant to relatively high doses of opioids and require even higher doses for acute severe pain. Similarly, people who are maintained on opioids for any reason become physically dependent and if their dose is abruptly ceased, they are likely to go into withdrawal. Opioid withdrawal may significantly worsen the experience of pain and may further complicate adequate pain management.

The physical conditions of tolerance and withdrawal do not in themselves indicate psychological dependence or problematic drug use. Definitions help to clarify the relationship among physical tolerance, dependence and pain management. Ranges of definitions are described in the following list. Some general principles and a number of common misconceptions follow these. Specific nursing guidelines are then described.

DEFINITIONS
Dependence
Physical dependence
Physical dependence occurs when the central nervous system (CNS) has been continually exposed to a drug and upon cessation of the drug the CNS goes into withdrawal. A rule of thumb is that the withdrawal syndrome will be the opposite of the drug's effects on the individual. For example, one of the withdrawal symptoms from a stimulant such as methamphetamine will be feelings of fatigue and possibly extended sleep. Withdrawal symptoms from a depressant such as alcohol or opioids will include agitation, sleep disruption and anxiety.

Psychological dependence
Psychological dependence is when someone has been continually exposed to a drug and upon cessation of the drug the person experiences psychological withdrawal. The person desires the drug and is preoccupied with thoughts of acquiring the drug. It may or may not be accompanied by the physical signs of withdrawal. Another definition (as well as another way to describe addiction) is the compulsion to use a drug despite knowledge that it is harmful. This process may occur with other non-drug forms of psychological dependence such as gambling or shopping.

Iatrogenic dependence
Iatrogenic dependence is where a person is treated with analgesics for a legitimate pain condition and subsequently develops a dependency. People suffering from painful conditions often express concern about this. They may state 'I need pain

relief but I don't want to become addicted' or even deliberately under-report their pain. However, iatrogenic dependency is uncommon following a single surgical procedure.

In some situations, iatrogenic dependence is more likely to occur. For example, an automobile accident may result in multiple traumas for a person. The person may be required to undergo a number of surgical procedures, resulting in a series of recovery periods with potentially inadequately managed pain.

The prospect of successive undermanaged pain episodes can be extremely stressful. It is more likely that the stress associated with the anticipation of undermanaged pain will be a trigger for the development of dependence than the effective use of opioids for pain management.

Pseudo-psychological dependence

Pseudo-psychological dependence, in the context of pain management, is where a person appears to be drug seeking but is merely trying to ensure adequate pain relief. The person may exhibit extremely inappropriate behaviour in their attempts to manage their pain.

They may be:
➤ involved in illegal activity such as buying opioids on the black market
➤ 'doctor shopping'
➤ displaying aggression
➤ stockpiling large amounts of opioids
➤ going to extreme lengths to manipulate professionals and friends to obtain opioids.

Psychological or pseudo-psychological dependence?

The differentiation between psychological dependence and pseudo-psychological dependence can be difficult for the professional.

KEY POINT 15.1

Adequate pain management is the key factor.

With adequate pain management, aberrant pseudo-psychological dependence behaviours should cease. If adequate pain management is provided and these behaviours do not cease then it is likely to be psychological dependence. The confounding factor is the difficulty in ascertaining if adequate pain management is being provided.[4] Failure to provide adequate pain management may increase the likelihood of progression to psychological dependence.[5]

Tolerance

Physical tolerance

Physical tolerance occurs when progressively larger amounts of the drug are required to get the same effect. Alternatively, if the amount of drug consumed remains constant, the effect of the drug diminishes. The development of physical tolerance by people on long-term opioid therapy is the central problem for effective pain management for this population. In spite of being maintained on relatively large amounts of opioids, individuals require even larger amounts of opioids for analgesic effect. Effective pain management starts by administering the dose usually required for an opioid-naïve individual and then titrating doses upwards until adequate pain relief is achieved. Analgesics should not be withheld unless the person is becoming oversedated.

Psychological tolerance

Psychological tolerance is when progressively larger amounts of the drug or addictive activity are required to get the same psychological effect. The person has got 'used to' the drug, the behaviour or the feelings experienced. For example, if the person has a gambling problem, they may feel the need to gamble more and more to derive the same sense of satisfaction they initially felt. This may occur without physiological changes.

A person's desired psychological effect from their drug of choice may be quite different from the prescriber's intended target therapeutic effect. Some people prefer to tolerate seemingly large amounts of pain with little analgesia. Others prefer to be sedated so that they feel only minimal discomfort. Just as the physiological perception of pain may differ among individuals, there is also a significant interpersonal variation in the psychological experience of pain. This is an important factor in a person's psychological tolerance.

Differential development of tolerance

Tolerance develops more rapidly to such effects as:
➤ analgesia
➤ euphoria
➤ sedation
➤ nausea
➤ vomiting
➤ respiratory depression.

Interestingly, it develops slowly or not at all to miosis (constriction of the pupils) and constipation. Those maintained on methadone and buprenorphine may complain of constipation for years after commencing treatment. Interestingly, opioid tolerance develops to the desired effects (e.g. analgesia and euphoria) as well as the undesired effects (e.g. opioid-related sedation and nausea).

Cross-tolerance

Tolerance to one opioid makes a person cross-tolerant to another opioid. It is the mechanism by which opioid substitution works. People are given long-acting methadone or buprenorphine because it stops the withdrawal syndrome associated with a shorter-acting opioid such as heroin. Similarly, benzodiazepines are administered to alcohol-dependent people to prevent them going into withdrawal (alcohol and benzodiazepines act at the same receptors and cross-tolerance occurs).

Pseudo-tolerance

Pseudo-tolerance in the context of acute pain management is where a person's level of use of a drug increases and they require an increased amount of opioid but it is not due to the development of analgesic tolerance.

It could be due to:

➤ drug interaction – if the person starts taking an additional drug, the analgesic drug may not be as effective
➤ progression of the disease or the development of a new disease
➤ increase in physical activity.

Hyperalgesia

> ### KEY POINT 15.2
>
> Pain is important for human functioning.

Pain signals to the brain that certain behaviour may cause injury. During opioid maintenance, there is a relatively large amount of opioid circulating around the body providing analgesia. The body, in an effort to provide homeostatic balance, becomes more sensitive to pain. It 'counterbalances' the analgesic effect of the opioid. Unfortunately, it commonly sensitises more than required and people maintained on opioids become more sensitive to pain, even those with high plasma opioid concentrations, compared with opioid-naïve people.

This may contribute to the development of opioid tolerance. As the body becomes more sensitive to pain, it requires more opioid to achieve a pain-free state. As stated, it is the primary complicating factor in the pain management of opioid-dependent people.

GENERAL PRINCIPLES

> ### KEY POINT 15.3
>
> There are misconceptions around the use of opioids, pain and dependence.

It is crucial that professionals have a good understanding of these general principles.

Maintenance opioids do not provide analgesia

There are three main factors preventing maintenance opioids from providing analgesia.

1 Methadone and buprenorphine have an analgesic duration of action of approximately 4–8 hours. Yet these drugs are administered and provide protection from withdrawal for 24–48 hours. Therefore, the period of pain relief is short relative to dosing periods.
2 Tolerance develops very rapidly to the analgesic effects of opioids when maintained for a period of time. The person becomes tolerant to both large amounts

of methadone or buprenorphine but is also cross-tolerant to the analgesic effects of other opioids.
3 The development of hyperalgesia.[4]

Adding opioids does not cause respiratory and CNS depression

As with analgesia, tolerance to the respiratory and CNS depression effects develops quickly. For example, as the pain increases for people with carcinomas, and opioid doses are increased in consequence, there is generally no increase in respiratory and CNS depression in doses adequate to achieve pain control. Pain is a natural antagonist to opioid-induced respiratory and CNS depression.

Seeking relief from pain is not the same as drug seeking

KEY POINT 15.4

Seeking relief from pain is different from drug seeking.

A careful clinical assessment for the objective evidence of pain will decrease the chance of manipulation by a drug-seeking person and also support the administration of opioid analgesics in a person with a history of drug dependence.

Professionals often perceive opioid-dependent people with pain issues to be demanding and manipulative. In turn, opioid-dependent people, often due to a history of discrimination and inadequate pain relief, may:
➤ become distrustful of the medical community and concerned about being stigmatised
➤ fear that their pain will be undertreated or that their opioid maintenance dose will be altered or discontinued
➤ act inappropriately to get opioids but only be suffering from unrelieved pain (pseudo-psychological dependence)
➤ have good pain relief but be fearful of the re-emergence of pain
➤ fear withdrawal symptoms should their pain relief be discontinued
➤ fear a reduction in the current effective doses of opioid analgesics.

Major health effects of unrelieved pain

KEY POINT 15.5

Major health implications are associated with unmanaged pain.

There are major health implications associated with unmanaged pain:
➤ physical stasis (bedsores, foot droop and so forth)
➤ prolonged postoperative recoveries
➤ clinical depression
➤ cardiovascular stress

> increased tumour growth
> relapse or exacerbation of dependence issues.

It is critical for pain to be managed to achieve optimal overall health.

Dangers associated with unrestricted opioid dosing

The answer is not as simple as dosing without restriction in an effort to produce pain relief. While there are dangers with unmanaged pain, there are dangers with unrestricted opioid dosing. While opioids theoretically have no maximum ceiling, hyperalgesia (as stated), neuroendocrinological (hormone) dysfunction and possibly immunosuppression (decreased functioning of the immune system) may occur at high doses. Respiratory depression can present difficulties in spite of tolerance (especially if the person is on other medication or consumes alcohol or another CNS depressant). Sedation can interfere with daily function and the processes of driving and safety around the home, and care of dependants may be affected with lethal consequences. It has also been suggested that repeated dose escalations lack incremental benefit at higher doses (e.g. more than 200 mg of morphine daily or equivalent).[1]

Factors affecting the pain experience

The pain experience of people maintained on opioids with chronic pain is not simply augmented by opioid-induced hyperalgesia. It is also exacerbated by subtle withdrawal syndromes. It may also be influenced by intoxication with related sympathetic arousal and muscle tension. Sleep disturbance, mood changes and functional changes (associated with a comorbid condition such as hepatitis C) may also affect the pain experience.[4,6]

Identifying and treating co-occurring conditions that affect the perception of pain, and, therefore, the successful management of the pain, is of paramount importance. Important examples of frequently comorbid conditions are depression and anxiety. Both may significantly complicate the treatment of pain and dependence, but may be responsive to a range of treatments.

SPECIFIC PAIN MANAGEMENT GUIDELINES FOR OPIOID-TOLERANT PEOPLE

People with active dependency

Build trust

> Openly acknowledge history of dependency and allow people to discuss fears about how this may affect pain management and treatment by the professionals.
> Reassure people that their history of dependency problems will not prevent adequate pain management.
> Respect and believe the person's report of pain.
> Reassure the person that professionals are committed to assertively providing effective pain relief.
> Aggressively treat acute pain; treatment for dependency issues is not the priority during the acute pain period.

Professional education

➤ Prescription of opioids to a person with a known dependency problem, for the management of pain, is not illegal or unethical.
➤ People with a dependency problem may be relatively pain intolerant.
➤ Detoxification is an ineffective short-term treatment for a dependency problem and inappropriate in the presence of pain.

Broaden the treatment plan

➤ With the person, develop a treatment contract for opioid analgesia.
➤ Request consultation from a substance use medicine specialist.
➤ Carefully document treatment plan, including analgesic use, response and regular reviews of efficacy of current plan.

Knowledgeably administer opioids

➤ Utilise non-pharmacologic and non-opioid analgesic alternatives.
➤ Consider patient-controlled analgesia, which may decrease total opioid requirements and the drug-seeking behaviours.
➤ Choose long-acting opioids (e.g. slow-release morphine sulphate; slow-release oxycodone) with gradual onset of action and lower street value, administered under continuous scheduled dosing orders (e.g. four times a day – QID) rather than as-needed orders (PRN).
➤ Opioid cross-tolerance and the person's increased pain sensitivity will often necessitate higher opioid analgesic doses administered at shorter intervals.

KEY POINT 15.6

If physically maintained on an agonist (e.g. methadone), **do not** administer a mixed opioid agonist/antagonist (e.g. buprenorphine) – withdrawal may be precipitated.[4]

Individuals on opioid maintenance therapy

➤ Continue the usual dose of methadone or buprenorphine (or equivalent).
➤ Use short-acting opioid analgesics and titrate to effect (e.g. morphine, codeine, oxycodone).
➤ Contact methadone or buprenorphine maintenance clinic or prescribing physician.
  — Notify them of admission, discharge and confirm the time and amount of last maintenance dose.
  — Notify them of any medications such as opioids or benzodiazepines given to the person during hospitalisation because they may show up on routine urine drug screening.
  — Notify them of any short-term analgesia (opioid or otherwise) provided on discharge.[4]

Individuals currently abstinent

Build trust

➤ Openly acknowledge a history of dependence and allow the person and professional to discuss fears of reactivation of dependency.

➤ Explain any intent to use opioids or other psychoactive medications.

➤ Respect the person's right to decide whether or not to be administered opioids.

Education of the individual

➤ Explain the health risks associated with unrelieved pain, including risk of relapse.

➤ Explain that the known risk for reactivation of dependency to opioids in the context of pain is small.

➤ Ensure the person understands the difference between psychological and physical dependence.

Minimise withdrawal following procedure or treatment

➤ Taper opioid analgesics **slowly** to minimise emergence of withdrawal symptoms.

➤ Assess for presence of withdrawal symptoms at least QID during analgesic taper; treat symptomatically.

➤ Offer non-pharmacological and non-opioid analgesic alternatives.

Support abstinence

➤ Encourage the person to increase contact with family and/or significant other supports. Reassure the person that it is acceptable to take medications for medical reasons. Offer to advise/reassure significant others if required.

➤ Request consultation from substance use medicine specialist.

➤ Request consultation from allied health professionals to devise pain management plans to support and minimise analgesic requirements.

➤ Screen for mental health and substance use conditions. Arrange diagnosis and treatment including referral if necessary.

➤ Include family in the plan of pain care.

➤ If relapse occurs, intensify abstinence efforts; do not terminate pain care.[4]

Individuals on naltrexone for alcohol or opioid dependence

➤ Cease naltrexone prior to pain-producing procedures if possible. Encourage the person to seek additional support as required to maintain abstinence during this period (3–5 days), and caution opioid-dependent individuals about the risk of inadvertent abstinence with relapse.

➤ In the initial 24-hour period as the naltrexone begins to wear off, the following multimodal analgesic regimes are recommended:
  – non-steroidal anti-inflammatories (e.g. ibuprofen)
  – paracetamol
  – ketamine

    — tramadol

    — regional nerve blocks/anaesthetics.

➤ **Caution:** There is experimental evidence of opioid receptor up-regulation following naltrexone/opioid antagonist withdrawal. Therefore, abrupt discontinuation of naltrexone may lead to increased opioid sensitivity and possibility of opioid toxicity with opioid administration. Increased supervision and monitoring is encouraged during this time.

➤ Continued administration of naltrexone will prevent the analgesic effects of regularly used doses of codeine- or opioid-based analgesia.

➤ If unable to decrease naltrexone (e.g. due to emergency department admission or for an emergency surgical procedure), the following multimodal analgesic regimes are recommended:

    — non-steroidal anti-inflammatories (e.g. ibuprofen)

    — paracetamol

    — ketamine

    — tramadol

    — regional nerve blocks/anaesthetics.

➤ If pain is not managed, people should be transferred to a high dependency unit and opioids titrated. At very high doses and in combination with opioid adjuvants . . .

    — non-steroidal anti-inflammatories (e.g. ibuprofen)

    — paracetamol

    — ketamine

    — tramadol

    — regional nerve blocks/anaesthetics

. . . opioids will override antagonist effects of naltrexone and provide relief. The therapeutic window may be narrow, necessitating careful monitoring for precipitous respiratory and CNS depression.[4]

Individuals experiencing chronic pain and dependence

➤ Complicated by the need to take opioids on a regular basis for the treatment of pain.

➤ Complicated by the lack of clear pathology underlying the pain experience.

➤ Complicated in that complete analgesia is not the practical goal of opioid treatment.

Treatment

➤ Address dependency issues.

➤ Use specific treatment contracts that should detail frequency of review, dispensing agreements and any specific monitoring.

➤ Define and manage physical and emotional components of pain. A range of interventions including counselling may be helpful. These might be particularly important if the painful condition has caused significant life changes or loss of function, resulting in grief and loss issues.

➤ Identify and treat mental health–substance use conditions as indicated.

➤ Provide holistic care including the use of physiotherapy and occupational therapy as required, addressing pain management and functional capacity. Interventions may include:
  − acupuncture
  − exercise plans
  − anxiety management
  − mindfulness training.

Assess, monitor and document
➤ Assess, monitor and document:
  − pain severity and quality
  − level of function
  − presence of adverse events
  − opioid analgesic use
  − evidence of opioid misuse
  − evaluation and plan
  − progress towards therapeutic goals.[7]

Therapeutic goals
➤ Include the functional restoration of:
  − physical capabilities
  − psychological intactness
  − family and social interactions
  − degree of healthcare utilisation
  − drug use for symptom control.[4]

Preparing for discharge
➤ If the individual has become dependent or remains dependent, minimise withdrawal.
➤ If already physically dependent on opioids, initiate long-acting substitute medications to prevent withdrawal.
➤ If detoxification prior to discharge is agreed upon, taper opioids **slowly** to minimise the emergence of withdrawal symptoms.
➤ Monitor for emergence of withdrawal symptoms at least QID, and treat aggressively and symptomatically.
➤ If discharged on opioid analgesics with limited maintenance:
  − choose a single, long-acting formulation with low street value (e.g. methadone or long-acting morphine)
  − prescribe decreasing quantities of opioids for short periods of time with no repeats. Specify frequent dispensing. Clearly communicate discharge plans and medications to all community professionals.
  − specify dosing times (not PRN)
  − assess person's level of motivation for drug treatment and encourage entry into treatment.[4]

CONCLUSION

Dependency, for people receiving opioids for dependency treatment or chronic pain, produces changes on a neurophysiological, psychological and societal level. In particular, there are the neural changes of opioid tolerance and hyperalgesia. Physical dependence and tolerance are predictable consequences of frequent opioid exposure and alone do not indicate maladaptive behaviour.

As a result of tolerance, people maintained on opioids will receive less analgesia from a given dose than people who are opioid naïve. Tolerant people will require higher opioid doses to manage acute severe pain. Maintenance opioids do not provide pain relief.

Iatrogenic dependence and relapse of dependency may occur as a result of *effective* management of acute severe pain, but are more likely to occur with *suboptimal* management of pain. Suboptimal management of pain is also likely to produce a variety of pseudo-dependence behaviours in a person's effort to ensure adequate pain relief.

Good practice should demonstrate a sound understanding of the pharmacodynamics and pharmacokinetics of pain medication in the context of opioid maintenance to prescribe, monitor and assess pain effectively in this population. It is important that professionals do not allow concerns of being manipulated to cloud their judgement concerning the individual's pain experience and lead them to providing suboptimal acute severe pain management. Careful monitoring and aggressive pain management will reassure the person, facilitate both physical and psychological recovery, and ensure the most effective management of both pain and dependency issues.

POST-READING EXERCISE 15.1 (ANSWERS ON PP. 227–8)

Time: 30 minutes
Read the following case study carefully then answer the questions. All names are fictitious.

Case study
Lisa (38) has a long-standing history of amphetamine and heroin dependence. She has been on methadone maintenance treatment for the last three years. She fell last night and fractured her forearm on a coffee table. She was admitted to the hospital. In the morning, she began to become agitated and demanded the 150 mg of methadone she claims she has daily. However, her urine drug screen has come back negative for methadone but positive for amphetamines. Lisa is scheduled for surgery on her arm later on that day.

- Why might Lisa have become agitated and demanded methadone?
- What further information do you need and where might you find it?
- What should your approach be to her pain relief?
- How would you discuss your observations and further assess Lisa?

REFERENCES

1 Chou R, Fanciullo GJ, Fine PG, *et al.* Clinical guidelines for the use of chronic opioid therapy in chronic noncancer pain. *Journal of Pain.* 2009; **10**: 113–30.

2 Alford DP, Compton P, Samet JH. Acute pain management for patients receiving maintenance methadone or buprenorphine therapy. *Annals of Internal Medicine.* 2006; **144**: 127–34.

3 Athanasos P, Smith CS, White JM, *et al.* Methadone maintenance patients are cross-tolerant to the antinociceptive effects of very high plasma morphine concentrations. *Pain.* 2006; **120**: 267–75.

4 Compton P, Athanasos P, de Crespigny C. *Opioid Tolerance and the Effective Management of Acute Pain.* Sydney: Drug and Alcohol Nurses of Australasia Conference; 2006.

5 Schnoll SH, Weaver MF. Addiction and pain. *American Journal of Addiction.* 2003; **12** (Suppl. 2): S27–35.

6 Parish JM. Sleep-related problems in common medical conditions. *Chest.* 2009; **135**: 563–72.

7 Passik SD, Kirsh KL. The need to identify predictors of aberrant drug-related behavior and addiction in patients being treated with opioids for pain. *Pain Medicine.* 2003; **4**: 186–9.

TO LEARN MORE

- Stimmel B. *Pain and its Relief without Addiction: clinical issues in the use of opioids and other analgesics.* Birmingham, NY: Haworth Medical Press; 1997
- Smith H, Passik S. *Pain and Chemical Dependency.* New York: Oxford University Press; 2008.
- International Association for Pain and Chemical Dependency website: www.iapcd.org (accessed 24 January 2011).

ANSWERS TO POST-READING EXERCISE 15.1

Lisa might have become agitated due to having uncontrolled pain because of her fracture. Her pain may be uncontrolled due to lack of analgesia or inadequate analgesia. Lisa may also be experiencing emerging withdrawal syndrome from one or both of her drugs of dependence. Information from Lisa's methadone treatment provider is necessary. This will confirm her current dose and dosing schedule including information to confirm the last dose given and any takeaway doses. Information about observed dosing will help to establish the likelihood of diversion of Lisa's prescribed methadone.

Confirmation of the results of Lisa's most recent urine drug screen will also be useful. It is important to confirm the type of urine drug screen test that was performed when Lisa was admitted to hospital as not all standard screens will detect methadone. The hospital laboratory will provide this information. Any recent medication changes are important to be aware of as some medications may significantly alter the metabolism of methadone. A serum methadone level (blood test) may be useful in cases such as this.

After confirming Lisa's methadone treatment dose and establishing that she is currently taking her methadone, her regular dose should be given. This regular dose will not provide any analgesia for her acute pain. Intraoperative pain relief should be given as usual and short-acting opioids should be titrated to effect. Postoperatively, long-acting opioids should be given with short-acting agents titrated for breakthrough pain. Non-opioid pain relief should also be used and may remain as part of the treatment plan as opioid analgesia is reduced after the initial effects of the injury begin to settle.

Lisa may have been receiving takeaway doses of methadone and diverting these doses elsewhere. This would have resulted in a negative urine screen for methadone. If there is any doubt as to Lisa's compliance with her current methadone treatment (concern about potential diversion) overall dose may be reduced and given as a split dose. Short-acting analgesic agents should be titrated to effect. Consultation with her usual methadone treatment providers should be sought in this instance to promote restabilisation prior to discharge.

Lisa should be reassured that her pain will be treated. She should be told that it could sometimes be somewhat more complicated to treat pain in those on methadone maintenance treatment but that staff will not give up until her pain is adequately treated. An explanation of the relevance of her recent drug use history – including the illicit use of drugs and pharmaceuticals – should be given alongside reassurance that any information given will be used solely to optimise her treatment.

Useful chapters

The Mental Health–Substance Use series comprises six books. To develop knowledge and understanding, chapters are interlinked, building and exploring specific areas. It is hoped the following will help readers locate relevant chapters easily.

BOOK 1: INTRODUCTION TO MENTAL HEALTH–SUBSTANCE USE

BOOK 2: DEVELOPING SERVICES IN MENTAL HEALTH–SUBSTANCE USE

Useful contacts

Collated by Jo Cooper

Addiction Arena – www.addictionarena.com
Addiction Medicine – http://listserv.icors.org/SCRIPTS/WA-ICORS.
   EXE?A0=ADD_MED
Addiction Project, The – www.theaddictionproject.com
Addiction Rehabilitation Facilities – www.arf.org/isd/bib/mental.html
Addiction Technology Transfer Center (ATTC) Network– www.attcnetwork.org
Addiction Today – www.addictiontoday.org
ADDICT-L List – http://listserv.kent.edu/archives/addict-l.html
Alcohol and Alcohol Problems Science Database – http://etoh.niaaa.nih.gov
Alcohol and Drug History Society – http://historyofalcoholanddrugs.typepad.com
Alcohol Concern (64 Leman Street, London E1 8EU, UK; Tel: 020 7264 0510;
   Fax: 020 7488 9213; Email: contact@alcoholconcern.org.uk) – www.alcoholconcern.
   org.uk/servlets/home
Alcohol Drugs and Development – www.add-resources.org
Alcohol Focus Scotland – www.alcohol-focus-scotland.org.uk
Alcohol Misuse (Department of Health) – www.dh.gov.uk/en/Publichealth/
   Healthimprovement/Alcoholmisuse/index.htm
Alcohol Misuse List – www.jiscmail.ac.uk/lists/ALCOHOL-MISUSE.html
Alcohol, Other Drugs, and Health: current evidence – www.bu.edu/
   aodhealth/index.html
Alcohol Policy Network – www.apolnet.ca
Alcohol Reports – www.alcoholreports.blogspot.com
Alcoholics Anonymous – www.aa.org
Alcoholism and Substance Abuse Providers – www.asapnys.org
American Association of Colleges of Nursing. *Tool Kit for Cultural Competent*
   Baccalaureate Nurses; 2008. (This site will soon have a toolkit for graduate education
   as well.) – www.aacn.nche.edu/Education/pdf/toolkit.pdf
American Psychiatric Association – www.psych.org
American Society of Addiction Medicine – www.asam.org/CMEonline.html
Australasian Professional Society on Alcohol and other Drugs – www.apsad.org.au
Australian Drug Foundation – www.adf.org.au
Australian Drug Information Network – www.adin.com.au

Australian Government Department of Health and Ageing:
  Alcohol – www.alcohol.gov.au
  Illicit drugs – www.health.gov.au/internet/main/publishing.nsf/content/
    healthpubhlth-strateg-drugs-illicit-index.htm
  Mental health publications – www.health.gov.au/internet/main/publishing.nsf/
    Content/mental-pubs
Berman Institute of Bioethics – www.bioethicsinstitute.org
Best Practice Portal – www.emcdda.europa.eu/best-practice
BioMed Central – www.biomedcentral.com
Brain Injury Australia – www.bia.net.au
Brain Trauma Foundation – www.braintrauma.org
Brief Addiction Science Information Source (BASIS) – www.basisonline.org
Campaign for Effective Prevention and Treatment of Addiction –
  www.solutionstodrugs.com
CASA: the National Centre on Addiction and Substance Abuse –
  www.casacolumbia.org
Centre for Addiction and Mental Health – www.camh.net
Centre for Clinical and Academic Workforce Innovation (Tel: 01623 819140; Email:
  ccawi@lincoln.ac.uk) – www.lincoln.ac.uk/ccawi
Centre for Evidence-based Mental Health (CEBMH) – www.cebmh.com
Centre for HIV and Sexual Health, Sheffield Primary Care NHS Trust – www.
  sexualhealthsheffield.nhs.uk
Centre for Independent Thought – www.centerforindependentthought.org
Centre for Mental Health – www.centreformentalhealth.org.uk
Clan Unity – www.clan-unity.co.uk
Clifford Beers Foundation. *Promotion of Mental Health*, vol. 1 (1992) – www.
  cliffordbeersfoundation.co.uk/jcont91.htm
Committee on Publication Ethics – http://publicationethics.org
Communities of Practice for Local Government – www.communities.idea.gov.uk
Community Nursing Network – www.communitynursingnetwork.org
Co-morbid Mental Health and Substance Misuse in Scotland – www.scotland.gov.uk/
  Publications/2006/06/05104841/0
Co-occurring Centre for Excellence (US) – www.coce.samhsa.gov
*Co-occurring Mental and Substance Abuse Disorders: a guide for mental health planning
  and advisory councils* (2003) – www.namhpac.org/PDFs/CO.pdf
Creative Commons – http://creativecommons.org
Cultural Competency in Health: a guide for policy, partnership and participation (2005) –
  www.nhmrc.gov.au/publications/synopses/hp25syn.htm
Daily Dose: drug and alcohol news from around the world. (This website is no longer in
  continuous service, but the archives are still available.) – http://dailydose.net
Dartmouth Psychiatric Research Centre – http://dms.dartmouth.edu/~prc
Department of Health – www.dh.gov.uk
Department of Primary Health Care – www.primarycare.ox.ac.uk/research/dipex
Doctors.net.uk – www.doctors.net.uk
Double Trouble in Recovery – http://doubletroubleinrecovery.org
    A list of peer-reviewed journal articles on Double Trouble in Recovery: http://
      doubletroubleinrecovery.org/research.html

Citations for biomedical literature published in peer-reviewed journals. Most citations resulting from a search for Double Trouble in Recovery link to the full text article: www.ncbi.nlm.nih.gov/pubmed

Drink and Drugs News – www.drinkanddrugs.net

Drinks Media Wire – www.drinksmediawire.com

Drug and Alcohol Findings – http://findings.org.uk

Drug and Alcohol Nurses of Australia – www.danaonline.org

Drug and Alcohol Services South Australia – www.dassa.sa.gov.au

Drug Day Programmes list – http://health.groups.yahoo.com/group/drug_day_programmes

DrugInfo Clearinghouse – http://druginfo.adf.org.au

Drug Misuse Information Scotland – www.drugmisuse.isdscotland.org

Drug Misuse Research list – www.jiscmail.ac.uk/lists/DRUG-MISUSE-RESEARCH.html

Drugs and Mental Health –www.thesite.org/drinkanddrugs/drugsafety/drugsandyourbody/drugsandmentalhealth

Drug Talk list – http://lists.sublimeip.com/mailman/listinfo/drugtalk

Drugtext Internet Library – www.drugtext.org

Dual Diagnosis – www.hoseahouse.org/infirmary/dualdx.html

Dual Diagnosis: Australia and New Zealand – www.dualdiagnosis.org.au

Dual Diagnosis Toolkit – www.rethink.org/dualdiagnosis/toolkit.html

Dual Diagnosis Website – http://users.erols.com/ksciacca

Enter Mental Health – www.entermentalhealth.net

European Alcohol Policy Alliance – www.eurocare.org

European Association for the Treatment of Addiction – www.eata.org.uk

European Federation of Nurses Associations – www.efnweb.org

European Monitoring Centre for Drugs and Drug Addiction – www.emcdda.europa.eu

European Working Group on Drugs Oriented Research – www.dass.stir.ac.uk/old-site/sections/scot-ad/ewodor.htm

Evidence-based Practice websites – http://davisplus.fadavis.com/purnell/evidence_based_weblinks.cfm

Eye Movement Desensitisation and Reprocessing Training Workshops – www.emdrworkshops.com

Faces and Voices of Recovery – www.facesandvoicesofrecovery.org

Federation of Drug and Alcohol Professionals – www.fdap.org.uk/certification/dap.html

Gambling International list – http://health.groups.yahoo.com/group/GamblingIssuesInternational/join?

Global Alcohol Harm Reduction Network – http://groups.google.com/group/gahrnet

Global Health Council – www.globalhealth.org

Guardian UK: the most useful websites on dual diagnosis – http://society.guardian.co.uk/mentalhealth/page/0,8149,688817,00.html

Headway – www.headway.org.uk

Health and Safety Executive (HSE) – www.hse.gov.uk/stress

HIT – www.hit.org.uk

Horatio: European Psychiatric Nurses – www.horatio-web.eu

Hub of Commissioned Alcohol Projects and Policies (HubCAPP). (This is an online resource of local alcohol initiatives throughout England and Wales.) – www.hubcapp.org.uk

Inexcess: in search of recovery – www.inexcess.tv

International Brain Injury Association – www.internationalbrain.org
International Centre for Alcohol Policies – www.icap.org
International Council of Nurses – www.icn.ch
International Council on Alcohol and Addictions – www.icaa.ch
International Drug Policy Consortium – www.idpc.net
International Harm Reduction Association – www.ihra.net
International Network of Nurses, The (TINN) – www.tinnurses.org
International Network on Brief Interventions for Alcohol Problems (INEBRIA) –
    www.inebria.net
International Nurses Society on Addictions – www.intnsa.org
International Society for the Study of Drug Policy – www.issdp.org
International Society of Addiction Journal Editors – www.parint.org/isajewebsite/
Intervoice: the International Community for Hearing Voices – www.intervoiceonline.org
IVO: scientific institute in lifestyle, addiction and related social developments –
    www.ivo.nl
James Lind Alliance Guidebook – www.jlaguidebook.org
James Lind Library – www.jameslindlibrary.org
Join Together: advancing effective alcohol and drug policy, prevention and treatment –
    www.jointogether.org
Madness and Literature Network – www.madnessandliterature.org
Management Standards Consultancy, The – www.themsc.org
Medical Council on Alcohol – www.m-c-a.org.uk
Medline Plus – www.nlm.nih.gov/medlineplus/dualdiagnosis.html
Mental Health (About.com) – http://mentalhealth.about.com
Mental Health and Addiction 101 (Centre for Addiction and Mental Health, Canada) –
    www.camh.net/MHA101/
Mental Health Europe – www.mhe-sme.org/en.html
Mental Health First Aid: Australia – www.mhfa.com.au
Mental Health First Aid: Canada – www.mentalhealthfirstaid.ca
Mental Health First Aid: England – www.mhfaengland.org.uk
Mental Health First Aid: Hong Kong – www.mhfa.org.hk
Mental Health First Aid: Scotland – www.smhfa.com
Mental Health First Aid: Singapore – www.mhfa.sg
Mental Health First Aid: South Africa – www.mhfasa.co.za
Mental Health First Aid: USA – www.thenationalcouncil.org/cs/program_overview
Mental Health First Aid: Wales – www.mhfa-wales.org.uk
Mental Health Forum – www.mentalhealthforum.net/forum
Mental Health Foundation – www.mentalhealth.org.uk
Mental Health in Higher Education – www.mhhe.heacademy.ac.uk/sitepages/
    educators/?edid=239
Mental Health Information for All (RCPSYCH) – www.rcpsych.ac.uk/
    mentalhealthinfoforall.aspx
*Mental Health Policy Implementation Guide: dual diagnosis good practice
    guide* (2002) – www.dh.gov.uk/en/Publicationsandstatistics/Publications/
    PublicationsPolicyAndGuidance/DH_4009058
Mental Health Research Network – http://homepages.ed.ac.uk/mhrn
Mentor Foundation, The – www.mentorfoundation.org
Methadone Alliance Forum, The – www.m-alliance.org.uk/forum.html

Middlesex University Dual Diagnosis Courses – www.mdx.ac.uk/courses/postgraduate/
nursing_midwifery_health/index/aspx
MIND: for better mental health – www.mind.org.uk
Ministry of Justice: National Offender Management Service – www.justice.gov.uk/about/
noms.htm
Mood Disorders Association of Canada – www.mooddisorderscanada.ca
Motivational Interventions for Drugs and Alcohol misuse in Schizophrenia – www.
midastrial.ac.uk
Motivational Interviewing – www.motivationalinterview.org
National Alliance on Mental Illness (US) – www.nami.org
National Centre for Education and Training on Addiction Australia – www.nceta.flinders.
edu.au
National Comorbidity Initiative Australia – www.health.gov.au/internet/main/publishing.
nsf/Content/health-pubhlth-publicat-document-metadata-comorbidity.htm
National Consortium of Consultant Nurses in Dual Diagnosis and Substance Use – www.
dualdiagnosis.co.uk
National Drug and Alcohol Research Centre – http://ndarc.med.unsw.edu.au
National Drug Research Institute – http://ndri.curtin.edu.au
National Health Service – www.nhs.uk
National Health Service Litigation Authority – www.nhsla.com
National Institute for Health and Clinical Excellence (Midcity Place, 71 High Holborn,
London, WC1V 6NA, UK; Tel: 0845 003 7780; Fax: 0845 003 7784; Email: nice@nice.
org.uk) – www.nice.org.uk
National Institute of Mental Health – www.nimh.nih.gov
National Institute on Alcohol Abuse and Alcoholism (NIAAA) (5635 Fishers Lane, MSC
9304, Bethesda, MD 20892-9304, USA; Tel: 301-443-3860; Email: www.niaaa.nih.gov/
ContactUs.htm) – www.niaaa.nih.gov
National Institute on Drug Abuse, National Institutes of Health (6001 Executive
Boulevard, Room 5213, Bethesda, MD 20892-9561, USA; Tel: 301-443-1124; Email:
information@nida.nih.gov) – www.nida.nih.gov
National Treatment Agency for Substance Misuse – www.nta.nhs.uk
New Directions in the Study of Alcohol – www.newdirections.org.uk
New South Wales Health Dual Disorders resources – www.druginfo.nsw.gov.au/
illicit_drugs
NHS Institute for Innovation and Improvement – www.institute.nhs.uk
Nordic Council for Alcohol and Drug Research (NAD) – www.norden.org/en/
areas-of-co-operation/alcohol-and-drugs
O'Grady CP, Skinner WJ. *A Family Guide to Concurrent Disorders* (2007) – www.camh.
net/Publications/Resources_for_Professionals/Partnering_with_families/partnering_
families_famguide.pdf
Ontario Mental Health and Addictions Knowledge Exchange Network – www.
ehealthontario.ca/portal/server.pt?open=512&objID=1398&PageID=0&mode=2
Oxford Centre for Neuroethics – www.neuroethics.ox.ac.uk
Partnership in Coping – www.pinc-recovery.com
Progress: National Consortium of Consultant Nurses in Dual Diagnosis and Substance
Use – www.dualdiagnosis.co.uk
Promoting Adult Learning – www.niace.org.uk/current-work/area/mental-health
Psychiatric Nursing – www.citypsych.com/index.html

Psychminded – www.psychminded.co.uk
Public Access (National Institutes of Health) – http://publicaccess.nih.gov/index.htm
Recovery Workshop – www.recoveryworkshop.com
Rethink (UK) – www.rethink.org/dualdiagnosis
Royal College of General Practitioners – www.rcgp.org.uk
Royal College of Psychiatrists – www.rcpsych.ac.uk
Royal College of Psychiatrists. *Changing Minds Campaign* – www.rcpsych.ac.uk/
   campaigns/previouscampaigns/changingminds.aspx
Royal Society for the encouragement of Arts, Manufactures and Commerce (RSA) –
   www.thersa.org
Sacred Space Foundation – www.sacredspace.org.uk
SANE Australia – www.sane.org
Schizophrenia Society of Canada – www.schizophrenia.ca
Scholarship Society – www.scholarshipsociety.org
Scottish Addiction Studies – www.dass.stir.ac.uk/sections/showsection.php?id=4
Scottish Addiction Studies Library – www.drugslibrary.stir.ac.uk
Social Care Institute for Excellence – www.scie.org.uk
Social Care Online – www.scie-socialcareonline.org.uk
Society for the Study of Addiction – www.addiction-ssa.org
Spanish Peaks Mental Health Centre – www.spmhc.org
Stigma in Mental Health and Addiction – www.cmhanl.ca/pdf/Stigma.pdf
Substance Abuse and Mental Health Center toolkit for integrated treatment for co-
   occurring disorders – http://mentalhealth.samhsa.gov/cmhs/CommunitySupport/
   toolkits/cooccurring
Substance Abuse and Mental Health Data Archive – www.icpsr.umich.edu/SAMHDA
Substance Abuse and Mental Health Services Administration – www.samhsa.gov
Substance Misuse Management in General Practice – www.smmgp.org.uk
Therapeutic Communities list – www.jiscmail.ac.uk/lists/
   THERAPEUTICCOMMUNITIES.html
Think Cultural Health: bridging the healthcare gap through cultural competence
   continuing education. (This site, developed by the US Department of Minority
   Health, has continuing education modules for physicians, nurses and other healthcare
   providers, and the Health Care Languages Implementation Guide.) – www.
   thinkculturalhealth.org and https://hclsig.thinkculturalhealth.hhs.gov
Tidal Model – www.tidal-model.com
Tilburg University, Department of Tranzo – www.uvt.nl/tranzo
Toc H – www.toch-uk.org.uk
Treatment Improvement Exchange – www.treatment.org
Trimbos Institute: Netherlands Institute on Mental Health and Addiction –
   www.trimbos.org
Turning Point – www.turning-point.co.uk
Tx Director – www.txdirector.com
UK Database of Uncertainties about the Effects of Treatment – www.library.nhs.uk/
   DUETs/Default.aspx
UK Drug Policy Commission – www.ukdpc.org.uk
UNGASS: United Nations General Assembly Special Session on the World Drug Problem
   – www.ungassondrugs.org
United Nations Office on Drugs and Crime – www.unodc.org

University of Toronto Joint Centre for Bioethics Centre for Addiction and Mental Health Bioethics Service – www.jointcentreforbioethics.ca/partners/camh.shtml

Update: an alcohol and other drugs information bulletin board – http://lists.sublimeip.com/mailman/listinfo/update

US Department of Health and Human Services. *Co-occurring Mental and Substance Abuse Disorders: a guide for mental health planning and advisory councils* (2003) – www.namhpac.org/PDFs/CO.pdf

Victorian Alcohol and Drug Association – www.vaada.org.au

Web of Addictions: links to other websites related to addiction – www.well.com/user/woa/aodsites.htm

Wired In to Recovery: empowering people to tackle substance use problems – http://wiredin.org.uk

World Health Organization: climate change and human health – www.who.int/globalchange/en

World Health Organization: management of substance abuse – www.who.int/substance abuse/en

World Health Organization: mental health – www.who.int/mental_health/policy/en

World Medical Association – www.wma.net/en/10home/index.html

Youth Drug Support, Australia – www.yds.org.au

Youth Health Talk – www.youthtalkonline.com

Index

Page numbers in **bold** indicate figures and tables.